Holistic Health Desk Reference

Natural Solutions to Mind-Body-Spirit Wellness

CW01574741

Dawn Grey, PhD, ND

The Holistic Health Desk Reference
Natural Solutions for Mind-Body-Spirit Wellness
Dawn Grey, PhD, ND

Visit our website at **www.reikiraysinstitute.com**

Library of Congress Cataloging-in-Publication Data

ISBN-13: 978-1461014010

ISBN-10: 1461014018

Printed in the United States of America

Table of Contents

Introduction

Many believe that today's modern medicine is traditional medicine. They have been raised to believe that trips to the doctor should result in the receipt of prescriptions and the consumption of antibiotics or other prescriptions for whatever ails them. I am here to tell you that allopathic medicine, treating the symptoms without discovering the root cause, is not traditional medicine.

I am not here to preach any one method of health and healing, nor do I offer this book as the be all and end all of medicine. I offer no promises of cures or miracles, and I certainly would not, even if the law allowed it, declare myself the keeper of some hidden secret of immortality. However, after years of research, study, and my own and other's turnaround in physical, emotional, and spiritual health, I firmly believe that there is far more to healing than masking a symptom.

Traditional medicine, as found in almost every culture's ancient Scriptures and practices, is highly effective at preventing disease and expediting health. As our world is shunning our consumerism and returning to a planetary awareness, the old ways of health are returning with a vengeance.

Ultimately, my goal is to empower the reader and client with the knowledge that choices exist. You need to be an active party in your health and wellness. The importance of diet, exercise, sleep, clean water, and hygiene, in conjunction with any or all of these modalities can greatly improve the quality of your life.

As such, the Holistic Health Desk Reference is a comprehensive guide to the betterment of your life and the world that we live in. I explain not only the natural remedies you can select, but how to perform these modalities on yourself and others, making this a teach-yourself manual and reference guide in one.

Dawn Grey, PhD, ND

Aromatherapy

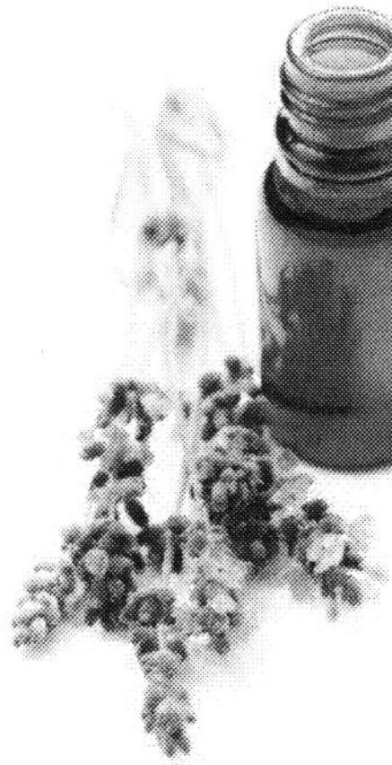

What is Aromatherapy?

Aromatherapy is the inhalation and application of essential oils from aromatic plants, grasses, bark, roots, trees, and flowers to restore or enhance health and beauty. It produces physical, spiritual, emotional, and mental sense of well-being. The principle of Aromatherapy is to strengthen the self-healing processes by preventative methods and indirect stimulation of the immune system. Aromatherapy is an ancient and popular approach to total well-being that is in tune with nature. Essential oils have been effectively used around the world for centuries for therapeutic purposes such as fighting infection, strengthening the immune system, reducing emotional and mental stress and providing a basis for preventative medicine.

A Brief History

We know from pictures on the walls of caves in France that aromatherapy has been in practice since at least 10,000 BC. In ancient Egypt, aromatherapy was a way of life. The scents of specific plants were used during religious rituals, because certain smells were believed to raise higher consciousness. Incense is still used in services of all religions today. Hypocrites, known as the Father of Medicine, was the first to study the cause and effect of aromatherapy. These studies led him to believe that daily aromatic baths and scented massages would promote good health. Holistic practitioners today follow the same belief. As people migrated across Europe, they carried with them the knowledge of benefits of specific herbs and oils of their native lands. The Renaissance and the expeditions of the great explorers gave way to new aromas. The twentieth century has brought a new enlightenment to this ancient art. During the turn of the century, French chemist and author, Dr. Gattefosse, brought a renewed interest in Aromatherapy. He discovered that different applications had antiseptic, anti-inflammatory, and antiviral effects. He experimented with these discoveries on soldiers during World War I. Today, a number of researchers and essential oil companies are doing their own experiments on how essential oils can help improve immunity and fight disease.

What Are Essential Oils?

Essential oils are highly concentrated extracts of flowers herbs, grasses, shrubs, and trees. These tiny droplets are found in particular glands, hairs or specific structures of the plant and contain the active principles, phytochemicals. Non-oily in texture, these highly concentrated substances are obtained by steam distillation, peel pressure, and solvent extraction methods. Only the highest quality pure essential oils have these medicinal properties—synthetics and fragrance oils do not. Read all labels carefully to make sure that you are receiving pure undiluted essential oils. Do research into brand names and get to know your local holistic shops for references.

How Do Essential Oils Work?

Essential oils work in harmony with the body to balance. They produce certain effects that we can count on, but can also adapt to the needs of different people. Used for their renowned anti-microbial and antiseptic effects, essential oils are not only safer than synthetic antibiotics but also support life (eubiotic) by working with the body's own natural healing abilities. Certain oils, such as Roman chamomile, have cytophylactic (cell regeneration) as well as antiseptic properties, making them the ultimate active principles for holistic natural skincare.

Oils can directly affect the physiological systems. Used topically for their antiseptic and soothing effects, essential oils can successfully treat minor skin conditions. It has been shown that the application of certain essential oils to the skin can produce vasodilation, which in turn causes warming of underlying muscles. In addition, because of the effect of relaxation on the brain and the subsequent sedating or stimulating of the nervous system, essential oils can also raise or lower blood pressure and possibly aid in normalization of hormonal secretion. Because essential oils have a direct connection to the brain, sending electrical messages directly into the limbic system, they can have effects on emotions and mental states. Perception of odors can have a major impact on memory, learning, and emotions. As therapeutic agents, essential oils work similar to tranquilizers but in a subtle, organic way. Most scents uplift spirits while at the same time calm the nervous system.

The sense of smell is 10,000 times more sensitive than any of the other senses. The human nose is capable of distinguishing between hundreds of thousands of different odors. Without the sense of smell, our capabilities to enjoy food or sex are greatly diminished. Smell is the only sense in which the receptor nerve endings are in direct contact with the outside world. The olfactory nerve is an extension of the brain itself, reached directly through the nose. This nerve is a direct link to our emotions, memory and learning. Essential oils trigger an olfactory nerve impulse, which goes directly to the brain and produces aromatherapy's far-reaching effects.

Essential oil vapors travel into the nose and interface with the olfactory epithelium, located at the top of each nostril. The olfactory epithelium consists of about 20 million nerve endings. One whiff of a scent triggers a nerve message to the brain, bringing with it an enormous amount of information. The olfactory bulb amplifies the message, which then passes to the limbic system, the part of the brain involved with emotions and memories. The amygdala and hippocampus are the first to analyze the nerve message. They are located in the part of the brain associated with memory, learning and emotional responses. At this point, a memory may be triggered because our subconscious receives and reacts to the nerve message before we actually think about what we smell. We use our intellectual processes when the nerve message is received by the cerebral cortex. Next, the message is passed on to the hypothalamus, which acts as a regulating or relay station that sends the message to several other parts of the brain. The thalamus, which is located in the center of the brain, triggers the release of neurochemicals called enkephalins. The pituitary gland, which is attached to the base of the brain, helps assist our aphrodisiac responses. It triggers the release of endorphins, which act as painkillers and can induce both euphoric and sexual feelings. The pituitary gland acts as the master endocrine gland governing all hormonal functions of the body, including the thyroid gland, the adrenals and the sexual glands. The raphe nucleus, which is located down the seam of the brain, helps assist our sedative responses. It triggers the release of serotonin, which has a relaxing and calming effect. Finally, the locus cereleus is responsible for our stimulant responses. It triggers the release of energizing noradrenaline into the brain. And believe it or not-- all of this begins to happen within seven seconds.

How To Use: Massage and Bodywork

Massage is one of the most effective methods of using the oils, combining their properties with the therapeutic power of touch. The oils should be diluted with an odorless carrier oil, such as grapeseed, sweet almond, jojoba or peach kernel. A dilution of 3% essential oil to carrier oil is a recommended starting point (less if using on sensitive skin or babies). This is approximately 1-6 drops of essential oil in two teaspoons of oil. Swedish Massage is the most popular massage used with aromatherapy because the stroking and kneading of the body stimulates the metabolism. Its active movements of the joints promote general relaxation, improve circulation and range of motion, and relieve muscle tension. Swedish massage is often given as a complete, full body technique, though sometimes only a part of the body is worked on.

Another method is Acupressure, which is finger pressure massage. Applying pressure to a pattern of specific points that correspond with the acupuncture points can help alleviate headaches and body tension. Pressure is applied with the thumb, finger, and palm rather than needles. The goal is the efficient and balanced flow of *chi* through the meridians. It is believed that where there is tension being held in the musculature, the flow of *chi* is impaired through those areas, which can lead to chronic problems not only in the musculature but also in the associated organs.

Spiritual/Energetic Aromatherapy

Energetic, or Spiritual Aromatherapy, is the practice of using the aroma of the oil to help stimulate a desired outcome. As such energetic aromatherapy can be performed distantly in addition to, or instead of other distance healing practices such as Reiki. This very simple method is utilized by selecting the oil or oils that correspond with the condition. The practitioner will either apply oils to a picture of the client, or apply the oils to his/her own body serving as the proxy for the client. Another way to use Energetic aromatherapy without having to anoint oils is to open the bottle and visualize the client being infused with its scent. You can also anoint gemstones with the oils and then arrange in a grid or layout that corresponds to the condition being worked on. Ultimately, spiritual aromatherapy works on intention, with the user intending for a condition to be alleviated, and using the proper visualization, affirmations, or supportive work to help manifest results.

How to Anoint With Oil

Sacred Oil can be used in a variety of different ways. Placing drops of the oil on places that hurt or symbolic points, such as your wrists and palms, symbolize the cleansing, purity, and sanctity of Christ or other religious figures. You can use diluted essential oil(s), or plain olive oil. Traditional scented anointing oils include frankincense, myrrh, and sandalwood.

Allowing someone else close to you to anoint your pressure points can be very helpful as it is sometimes difficult to detect your own power centers. Having someone anoint you can help you to relax and open yourself to the healing and benefits of the oil and aromatherapy.

Anointing yourself can also be a daily self-practice or type of meditation that you use to focus energy and healing into your chakras and power centers.

Some religious practices only allow higher up clergy or members use this practice. Depending on your view and use of the oil, you can tailor it to your personal uses.

Martial artists often anoint themselves and their power points with oil to help with awareness, alertness, and balance their chi during fights.

Emotional Uses of Aromatherapy

Condition	Suggested Oils
Aggression	Bergamot, Chamomile, Juniper, Lemon, Marjoram, Rosemary, Ylang Ylang
Anger	Chamomile,Jasmine,Marjoram, Palma Rosa,Rose, Rosemary,Ylang-Ylang,
Anxiety	Neroli, Bergamot, Chamomile, Frankincense, Geranium (for balance), Lavender, Orange, Patchouli, Rose (for confidence), Sandalwood. Sweet Marjoram, Vetiver (for grounding)
Disappointment	Bergamot, Cypress, Frankincense, Jasmine, Orange, Rose
Fear	Cedarwood, Fennel, Ginger, Patchouli, Sandalwood, Thyme
Grief	Bergamot, Chamomile, Jasmine, Marjoram, Neroli, Rose
Hysteria	Chamomile, Lavender, Neroli, Orange, Tea Tree
Impatience	Chamomile, Clary, Frankincense, Lavender
Indecision	Basil, Clary, Cypress, Jasmine, Patchouli, Peppermint
Jealousy	Jasmine, Rose
Loneliness	Benzoin, Marjoram
Fatigue(emotional and mental	Basil, Clary Sage, Cardamom, Cinnamon Leaf or Bark, Clove bud, coriander, Eucalyptus Citriodora, Ginger, Grapefruit, Helichrysum, Jasmine, Juniper, Orange, Palmarosa, Peppermint, Rosemary, Thyme, Vetiver, Ylang Ylang
Fatigue (physical)	Basil, Elemi, Ginger, Lemon, Lavender, Orange, Peppermint, Rosemary
Nervousness	Chamomile, Clary, Coriander, Frankincense, Neroli, Orange, Vetiver
Panic	Chamomile, Clary, Geranium, Jasmine, Juniper, Lavender, Neroli, Ylang Ylang
Sadness	Benzoin, Jasmine, Rose, Rosewood
Shock	Lavender, Neroli, Rose, Teatree
Shyness	Black Pepper, Ginger, Jasmine, Patchouli, Peppermint, Rose, Neroli, Ylang Ylang
Stress	Bergamot, Atlas Cedarwood, Roman Chamomile, all Citrus oils, Clary Sage, Frankincense, Geranium, Lavender, Sweet Marjoram, Melissa, Neroli, Patchouli, Petitgrain, Rose (absolute and otto), Rosemary, Sandalwood, Vetiver, Ylang Ylang.
Suspicion	Jasmine, Lavender
Tension	Chamomile, Clary, Cypress, Frankincense, Geranium, Jasmine, Lavender, Lemon, Marjoram, Neroli, Orange, Rose, Rosewood, Sandalwood, Ylang Ylang

Physical Ailments and Suggested Oils

Allergies:	Blue Tansy, German and Roman Chamomile, Helichrysum, Lavender, Yarrow.
Asthma:	Blue Tansy, Frankincense, Hyssop, Ravensara, Cedarwood, Cajeput, Clary Sage, Roman Chamomile, Cypress, Fennel, Eucalyptus Radiata, Hyssop, Lavender, Pine, Lemon, Mandarin, Myrtle, Peppermint, Petitgrain, Rosemary.
Arthritis	Lavandin, Helichrysum, Black Pepper, Ginger, Marjoram, Lavender, Lemon, Nutmeg, Rosemary, Cajeput, Cinnamon, Clove Bud, Eucalyptus, Angelica Seed, Roman Chamomile, Holy Basil, Clove Bud, Cypress Tips, Balsam Fir, Juniper, Nutmeg, Dalmatian Sage, Thyme, Wintergreen.
Athletes Foot and fungal infections.	Myrrh, Patchouli, Lemongrass, Niaouli, Palma Rosa, Tagetes, Tea Tree.
Backaches	Helichrysum, Lavandin, Black Pepper, Cajeput, Chamomile, Eucalyptus, Ginger, Juniper Berry, Lavender, Lemon, Peppermint, Marjoram, Nutmeg, Rosemary, Thyme.
Boils:	Bergamot, Lavender, Lemon, Tea Tree, Thyme, Juniper, Geranium (in hot compresses)
Bronchial Congestion:	Hyssop, Frankincense, Spruce, Copaiba Balsam, Balsam Fir, Pine.
Bruises:	Helichrysum, Black Pepper, German Chamomile, Hyssop, Fennel, Lavender, Lemon, Rosemary.
Burns:	Lavender, Helichrysum, Carrot Seed, Frankincense, Manuka, Neroli, Tea tree.
Candida (Yeast Infection)	Tea tree, Cajeput, Holy Basil, Melissa, German Chamomile, Lemon Eucalyptus.
Chronic Fatigue	Sweet Basil, Rosemary, Geranium, Lemon, Grapefruit.
Chronic Pain	**Topical Application:** Black Pepper, Clove bud, Frankincense, Ginger, Juniper, Lavender, Lemongrass, Sweet Marjoram, Myrrh, Peppermint, Rose, Rosemary, Ylang Ylang. **Inhalation:** Frankincense, Lavender, Lemongrass, Sweet Marjoram, Rosemary, Lemon Verbena.

Cold Sores (Herpes simplex):	Melissa, Rose, Myrrh, Bergamot, Eucalyptus Globulous, Sandalwood, Bergamot, Eucalyptus Radiata, Cajeput, Niaouli, Ravensara, Tea Tree.
Congestion (chest and bronchial)	Eucalyptus Globulous, Sweet Eucalyptus, Frankincense, Sweet Basil, Black Pepper, Lemon Myrtle, Peppermint, Pine, Spruce.
Constipation:	Fennel, Yarrow, Black Pepper, Marjoram, Rosemary, Carrot Seed, Peppermint, Pine, Orange.
Coughs	Hyssop, Cardamom, Balsam Fir, Pine, Sage, Oregano, Eucalyptus.
Cramps, Muscle Spasms	Marjoram, Black Pepper, Roman Chamomile, Clary Sage, Cypress, Geranium, Lavender, Marjoram, Thyme.
Cuts and scrapes	Lavender, Chamomile, Tea Tree, Helichrysum.
Cystitis	Bergamot, Atlas Cedarwood, Juniper, Cypress.
Dandruff	Tea tree oil, added to shampoo in a 5% dilution.
Diarrhea:	Black Pepper, German and Roman Chamomile, Cinnamon, Cypress, Eucalyptus, Sweet Fennel, Ginger, Mandarin, Neroli, Peppermint, Cajeput.
Edema	Cistus, Angelica, Ravensara, Rosemary, Carrot seed, Fennel, Grapefruit, Juniper, Lemon, Mandarin, Tangerine.
Fever	Sponge the body with cool water with 1 drop each Eucalyptus, Lavender, and Peppermint oils added.
Gas:	Massage onto body: Ginger, Peppermint, Anise Seed, Fennel, Litsea, Oregano, Black Pepper, Cardamom, Roman and German Chamomile.
Gout:	St. John's Wort oil as a carrier with 5% Wintergreen, Juniper Berry, Lemon, Rosemary.

Headaches:	Lavender, Sweet Basil, Roman Chamomile, Clove Bud, Lavandin, Cajeput, Clary Sage, Eucalyptus, Marjoram, Peppermint, Rosewood, Rosemary, Thyme.
Hot Flashes:	Vitex, Peppermint, Geranium.
Hypertension (High Blood Pressure):	Bergamot, Roman chamomile, Lavender, Litsea, Melissa, Marjoram, Neroli, Ylang Ylang.
Hypotension (Low Blood Pressure)	Ginger, Lemon, Red Thyme, Rosemary.
Indigestion	Cardamom, Black Pepper, Ginger, Peppermint, Anise Seed, Coriander, Fennel, Lemongrass, Litsea, Melissa, Nutmeg, Cinnamon Leaf, Sweet Fennel.
Inflammation	Helichrysum, Roman or German Chamomile, Coriander, Juniper, Fennel, Nutmeg, Yarrow.
Insect Bites	Cajeput, Helichrysum, German Chamomile, Lavender.
Insomnia	Red Mandarin, Lavender, Roman Chamomile, Clementine, Petitgrain, Bergamot, , Myrtle, Petitgrain, Sandalwood, Spikenard,Valerian.
Lymphodema	Cistus, Helichrysum, Lavender.
Menopause	Clary Sage, Geranium, Rose, Vitex, Bergamot, Chamomile, Cypress, Fennel, Jasmine, Neroli, Ylang Ylang.
Menstrual Cramps	Clary Sage, Sweet Marjoram, Geranium, Sweet Fennel, Parsley, Anise Seed, Sweet Basil, Roman Chamomile, Clary Sage, Cypress, Yarrow.
Migraines	Lavender, Peppermint, Roman Chamomile, Clary Sage, Marjoram, Valerian, Eucalyptus, Neroli.
Muscle Aches	Lavandin, Rosemary, Black Pepper, Ginger, Black Spruce, Sweet Basil, Lavender, Vetiver, Eucalyptus.
Muscle Spasms	Roman Chamomile, Petitgrain, Clary Sage, Fennel, Frankincense, Lavender, Sage.
Nausea	Ginger, Peppermint, Spearmint, Cardamom Seed, Sweet Fennel, Patchouli.

Peridontal problems	Myrrh, Sweet Fennel, Manuka, Peppermint, Tea Tree.
PMS	Geranium, Clary Sage, Rose, Sweet Fennel, Bergamot, Chamomile, Juniper Berry, Lavender, Neroli, Rosemary, Sweet Fennel, Palma Rosa, Rose Otto, Vitex, Ylang Ylang Extra,
Pressure sores (Bed Sores)	German Chamomile, Helichrysum, Geranium, Frankincense, Lavender, Calendula infused oil.
Rheumatism	St. John's Wort Oil, Black Pepper, Ginger, Helichrysum, Lavender, Lavandin, Wintergreen.
Scabies	Tea Tree(5% dilution) mixed in a carrier oil.
Sciatica	St. John's Wort Oil, Black Pepper, Ginger, Helichrysum, Lavender, Lavandin.
Sinuses	All Eucalyptus varieties, especially Radiata, Peppermint, Angelica Root, Sweet Basil, Clove Bud, Hyssop, Lemon, Lemon Myrtle, Pine.
Shingles:	Ravensara, Bergamot, Eucalyptus Globulous, Melissa with Rose Otto, Lavender, Tea Tree.
Sore Throat:	Hyssop, Sandalwood, Myrrh.
Sunburn	Chamomile with Lavender, Blue Tansy, German Chamomile, Peppermint.
Varicose Veins:	Calendula infused oil, Cypress, Lemon, Geranium, Juniper, Rosemary.

Aromatherapy Oil Recipes

Drop equivalent: 1-10 drops of oil to 1 tbsp.(15ml). Always use a carrier oil when using essential oils. Never use undiluted, which is also referred to as "Neat."

Pain Reliever:	***Calming/ Stress:***	***Communication:***
Eucalyptus 5 drops	Lavender 3 drops	Frankincense 4 drops
Pine 5 drops	Rosewood 3drops	Geranium 4 drops
	Sandalwood: 2 drops	Ylang Ylang 3 drops

Fatigue:	***Uplifting:***	***PMS:***
Bergamot 4 drops	Lemongrass 5 drops	Lavender 4 drops
Pine 4 drops		Ylang Ylang 4 drops
		Geranium 2 drops

Reflexology mix:	***Romance:***	***Headache:***
Peppermint 4 drops	YlangYlang 4 drops	Peppermint 5 drops
Lavender 4 drops	Patchouli 2 drops	Lavender 5 drops
Rosemary 2 drops	Orange 2 drops	

Relaxing/Calming Blends: Mix with 2 Tablespoons carrier oil.

Eucalyptus 2 drops	Cedarwood 3 drops	Lavender 3 drops
Spearmint 3 drops	Sage 2 drops	Palmarosa 2 drops

Uplifting Blends: Mix with 2 Tablespoons carrier oil

Grapefruit 3 drops	Orange 3 drops	Bergamot 3 drops
Peppermint 2 drops	Ginger 3 drops	Lavender 3 drops

Orange 3 drops	Peppermint 2 drops	Rosemary 2 drops
Patchouli 2 drops	Lavender 3 drops	Lime 4 drops

*** NOTE: if you are working on children dilute further*To make a mist, omit the oil and add to 4-oz water and double the recipe.**

Baths

Using oils in baths is simple, effective, and a pleasant way to relax and receive the therapeutic effects. Water has therapeutic value, which enhances the powers of the oils. To use, add 6 to 10 drops of essential oil, (or a blend), to the surface of the water which has already been run, then soak for about 20 minutes, while you inhale the vapor. (Again reduce the amount of oils used in baths for babies).

Compresses

Add 5 to 10 drops of essential oil to 1qt. of warm water. Then soak a piece of clean cloth in the water. Wring out and place the cloth on the affected part. When in doubt- use lavender, the most all purpose of all the oils.

Inhalation

Add 5 to 10 drops of essential oil into a bowl of steaming water, then place a towel over your head and the bowl and inhale the vapor for a few minutes. This is great for colds and sinus congestion.

Diffusion

All essential oils evaporate easily, so they make very good air-fresheners. Different oils create different atmospheres, so experiment! For example, relaxing Sandalwood or Clary Sage is good for nighttime; or Peppermint clears your mind when you need to work. There are many vaporizers out there from the simple bowl of water on the radiator with a few drops of oil on the surface, to light bulb rings and vaporizer bowls which sit above candleholders. There is even an effective electric vaporizer dispensing fragrance from a low heat source, thereby making the water and the oils last longer than usual.

Perfumes

Make your own perfume by blending different oils. Try experimenting with different combinations, which can be mixed with a carrier oil or lotion. This is fun and easy to do.

Skin Care

Here is a list of some of the oils that are good for different skin types. Choose one or more and dilute in the suggested carrier, or add to your favorite cleanser.

Normal skin:
Lavender, palmarosa, geranium, chamomile, rosewood, benzoin, mixed with hazelnut oil.

Dry skin:
Sandalwood, rosewood, lavender, patchouli, geranium, chamomile in jojoba, sesame or avocado oil.

Oily skin:
Ylang Ylang, lemon, lime, orange, lavender, juniper in a carrier of grapeseed oil.

Problem skin:
Myrrh, lavender, geranium, chamomile, sandalwood, rosewood in a carrier of almond oil.

Sunburn relief:
Lavender and peppermint in aloe vera gel.

Selecting and Storing Oils

Because essential oils are affected by sunlight they should be sold and stored in dark glass bottles, with tightly sealed caps. Make sure that the cap is on securely and the bottle stored upright in a cool dark place. The oils should be stored out of sight and the reach of children. Never store essential oils in plastic bottles. Good Essential oils should keep for several years if properly stored, though the oils of orange, lemon, and lime will not keep as long. Patchouli is at the other extreme and actually gets better as it ages. For quality, just remember, you get what you pay for. Some oils are naturally inexpensive, such as most citrus and tree oils, whereas florals are primarily costly. Jasmine, rose, and Melissa can be over $100 for 5ml so choose wisely—if you find jasmine for under $10, its either synthetic or diluted. Read labels and use your intelligence when making your purchases.

Essential Oils and Their Properties

Allspice (Pimento): Its aroma resembles a mixture of pepper, clove and cinnamon. This oil is stimulating and vitalizing. It has been used to treat depression, nervous exhaustion, arthritis, fatigue, stiffness, flatulence, and indigestion. Debatable whether it should be used in massage since it is such a powerful oil. May irritate the skin and mucous membranes. Very warming oil, gets the circulation going. Blends well with frankincense ginger lemon and orange.

Anise (Pimoinella anisum): Spicy, warm, licorice-like aroma. Well known for its effect on the digestive system. May have a good effect on asthma and breathing difficulties. Sexual problems such as impotence and frigidity may be helped. Said to control lice, good for infectious skin diseases. Blends well with fennel, petitgrain, and rosewood.

Balsam (Myroxylon pereirae): Also used as an anti-infective. Used on chafed skin to soothe. Exotic aroma, anchoring, strengthening and imparts a rich, earthy scent to perfumes. It is a skin sensitizer. Use with caution and apply a high SPF sunscreen up to 72 hours after use to reduce burn risk.

Basil, Sweet (Ocimum basilicum): Warm, fiery scent. Good for tired, overworked muscles, as a mouthwash for sores and infected gums (apply to areas, do not drink or swallow), for chest infections and digestive problems. Blends well with bergamot, lavender, neroli and verbena.

Bay (Larus nobilis): Light, spicy, sweet aroma. May act as an appetite stimulant and to settle stomach pains. General aches and pains, as well as rheumatic pains may be alleviated. Blends well with rose, cedarwood, and eucalyptus.

Benzoin (Styrax benzoin): Cinnamon-Vanilla like. It is warming to the body, reduces stress and is calming. Mood uplifting, breaks up congestion. Works well with Spicy scents.

Bergamot (Citrus bergamia): Uplifting, spicy, sweet scent; like orange and lemons with floral overtones. Inhaled, it relaxes the nervous system and acts as a digestive. Also known as an expectorant, antidepressant and antiseptic. Blends well with chamomile, lavender, neroli and geranium. Bergamot is a photosensitizer (increases the skin reaction to sunlight and makes it more likely to burn) and the effect can last for several days.

Birch, sweet (Betula alba): A powerful oil which could irritate sensitive skin. Best used with caution or not at all. Has an invigorating, even rousing effect on the spirits. Stimulates the sweat glands aiding the body in releasing harmful toxins. A lymphatic cleaner and helps keep infection at bay. Increases the flow of urine. Its diuretic properties could also help with obesity and cellulite. Could be good of rheumatism and muscle pain generally since it eliminates accumulation of uric acid in the joints. Blends well with chamomile, frankincense, and lemon.

Cajeput (Melaleuca leucadendron): Camphor fragrance. Relaxes muscles, relieves aches and pains. Good to use to treat the skin when apply henna tattoos. A good substitute for wintergreen.

Camphor (Cinnamomum camphora): Fresh, clean and very penetrating. Analgesic, antidepressant, antiseptic, antispasmodic, diuretic, stimulant, laxative and vermifuge. A very powerful oil, overdosing could cause convulsions and vomiting even if only applied to skin. Should be avoided in pregnancy and people suffering from epilepsy and asthma. Sedates nervy types particularly when associated with depression. Raises low blood pressure. Warms and cools the body where necessary. Good for constipation and diarrhea. Also helpful with gastroenteritis. May be helpful with stiff muscles. It is cooling on the skin and, therefore, reduces inflammatory conditions. Blends well with basil, and chamomile.

Carrot Seed (Daccus carota): Slightly sweet and dry aroma. Used to treat jaundice and other liver disorders. Recommended for mature skin and/or wrinkled skin. Blends well with bergamot, lemon, orange and rosemary.

Caraway (Carum carvi): Minty. Muscle relaxant relieves pain, improves digestion. Blends well with eucalyptus and rosemary.

Cardamom (Elettaria cardamomum): Spicy. Muscle relaxant, skin conditioner, soothing agent, stimulating, toning. Blends well with geranium, juniper berry and lemon.

Cassia (Cinnamomum cassia): Cinnamon-like aroma. Used to stimulate the pancreas. Blends well with all the spice and citrus oils, geranium and black pepper.

Cedarwood (Cedrus atlantica): Sweet woody aroma which improves as the oil ages; it is a dark, amber viscous liquid. Some of its properties are antiseptic, antiseborrheic, astringent, and aids in the removal of body fat. Used externally for cellulite. Blends well with bergamot, clary sage, frankincense, oakmoss and rosemary.

Celery (Apium graveolens): spicy, stimulating, toning. Great for gout and water retention. Blends well with basil, cajeput, lemon, orange, palmarosa, rosemary.

Chamomile, German and Roman (Matricaria chamomilla/Anthemis nobilis): Both have a fruity, apple-like aroma. Both contain Azuline, a powerful anti-inflammatory. German has slightly more and is a deeper blue color. Both have analgesic, antidepressant, and sedative properties. Blend well with bergamot, jasmine, rose, and ylang ylang.

Cinnamon, Cinnamon leaf (Cinnamonzeylanicum): Spicy, sharp, and sweet aroma. Used as an insecticide, antispasmodic and aphrodisiac. Eases colds and breathing difficulties, freshens breath. Very powerful, should be used with extreme care, skin irritant. Blends well with clove, frankincense, lavender, orange and thyme.

Citronella (Cymbopogon nardus): Slightly sweet and lemony aroma. Used as an insecticide and antidepressant. Its most useful quality seems to be as an insect repellant. May also help pets get rid of fleas. Also known to clear the mind so may be useful against headaches and migraines. Blends well with citrus oils, peppermint, and eucalyptus.

Clary Sage (Salvia sclarea): Heavy, herbal, nutty fragrance. A relaxing, warming oil, eases nervous tension. Hormone balancer, may regulate scanty periods. Also soothes digestive problems. Blends well with bergamot, lavender, lime, and geranium.

Clove (Eugenia caryophyllata): Clove has a spicy and penetrating aroma. Highly irritant to the skin, must be diluted. Beneficial to the digestive system, effective against diarrhea, vomiting and spasms. Can help toothache, rheumatism, arthritis and mouth sores. Blends well with basil, cinnamon, citronella, and orange.

Coriander (Coriandrum sativum): Slightly pungent, sweet and spicy aroma. Stimulates the mind, especially in the presence of fatigue and tension. May help memory. Relieves stomach gas and cramps. May have some effect on bad breath. Alleviates muscle spasms. Blends well with bergamot, lemon and jasmine.

Cypress (Cupressus sempervirens): Cypress has a woody and slightly spicy aroma. Its effect on varicose veins is well known. Regulates menstrual cycle. Soothes anger. Blends well with bergamot, lavender, lemon, pine and sandalwood.

Eucalyptus (Eucalyptus globulus): Woody, lemon aroma. Very effective insect repellent. Excellent decongestant. Blends with rosemary, peppermint, and lemon.

Fennel (Foeniculum vulgare): Floral, herby and slightly spicy aroma. It is antiseptic, diuretic, insecticide and laxative. It is an excellent body cleanser, may rid the system of toxins from alcohol and excessive eating, great for hangovers. Tonic to the digestion. Good for vomiting and colic. Antispasmodic, relieves colic, constipation and gas. Decreases appetite. Increases milk flow in nursing mothers. Blends well with lavender, lemon, rose, and sandalwood.

Fir Needle (Abies alab): Clear, balsamic, and refreshing aroma. It is antiseptic, expectorant and sedative. May have a beneficial effect on chest conditions, such as fluid and mucous. Helps with muscle aches. Blends well with basil, cedarwood and frankincense.

Frankincense (Boswellia thurifera): Woody, spicy, incense-like. It is antiseptic, diuretic, digestive and sedative. Very helpful in clearing the lungs. Eases shortness of breath. May diminish effects of cystitis and genito-urinary infections. May relieve heavy periods, acts as a tonic to the uterus. Soothes the stomach, eases belching. Blends well with basil, geranium, lavender, orange and sandalwood.

Geranium (Pelargonium graveolens): antidepressant, antiseptic, and insecticide. Calms anxiety and assists with depression. Useful with premenstrual tension. May assist with menopausal problems. Assists with breast inflammation. Helps clear the body of toxins. May be helpful with addictions. Stimulates the lymphatic system. Eases neuralgia. Blends well with basil, bergamot, carrot, jasmine, lavender and rose.

Ginger (Zingiber officinale): Spicy, woody, and warm, with a hint of lemon. It is antiseptic, analgesic, expectorant, laxative, and aphrodisiac. Aids memory. Eases sore throats. Settles the digestive system, effective against nausea, hangovers, jet lag, sea and travel sickness. Relieves cramps, rheumatic pains and muscle spasms. A valuable remedy in cases of impotence. Blends well with cajeput, cinnamon, eucalyptus, frankincense, geranium, orange and verbena.

Grapefruit (Citrus paradisi): Has a sweet, sharp, citrusy aroma. It is antidepressant, antiseptic, diuretic and disinfectant. Invaluable in times of stress uplifts and revives the spirit. May have an effect on obesity, fluid retention, and cellulite. It is a tonic to the liver. Breaks down fats and makes them easier to metabolize. May help lower cholesterol and triglycerides. Causes photosensitivity, so use sunscreen for 72 hours after topical application. Relieves migraine and premenstrual tension and jet lag. Blends well with bergamot, cedarwood, frankincense, and lavender.

Hyssop (Hyssopus officinalis): Warm, sweet, penetrating aroma. It is antirheumatic, antiseptic, antispasmodic, astringent, cicatrizing, digestive, diuretic, emmenagogue, expectorant, febrifuge, emollient, hypertensive, nervine, sedative, stimulant, stomachache, sudorific and vermifuge. This very potent oil is recommended in very low dosages. People suffering from epilepsy and high blood pressure should stay clear of it. Not to be used during pregnancy. Said to cure grief by clearing the spleen. Raises low blood pressure. Very effective on respiratory problems and viral infections Acts as a mild laxative, relieves stomach cramps, expels wind and is said to get rid of worms. Beneficial to the menstrual cycle, particularly with water retention during periods and effective against amenorrhoea. Blends well with fennel, lavender, and tangerine.

Jasmine (Jasminum sambac): Sweet, flowery, exotic aroma. Called the "king of flower oils" has a reputation as an aphrodisiac. It is antidepressant, antiseptic, emollient and sedative. Excellent for severe depression. Calms the nerves. Effective in postpartum depression. Promotes flow of breast milk. Relieves spasm of the bronchi, calms irritating coughs. Blends well with bergamot, frankincense, rose, orange and sandalwood.

Juniper (Juniperus communis): Refreshing and slightly woody aroma. It is antiseptic, antispasmodic, aphrodisiac, diuretic, and insecticide. Not to be used if you have any type of kidney or inflammatory problems. Effective diuretic and antiseptic of the genito-urinary tract, very valuable in treating cystitis and kidney stones. Helps with cellulitis. Clears intestinal mucous. Helpful in cases of gout and rheumatism as it helps to eliminate uric acid. Regulates period and eases painful cramps. Blends well with bergamot, cypress, frankincense, and sandalwood.

Lavender (Lavandula officinalis): It would take many pages to outline all the benefits and properties of lavender. It is analgesic, antidepressant, antirheumatic, antiseptic, antispasmodic, antiviral, bactericide, decongestant, deodorant, diuretic, fungicide, sedative. Soothes the spirit, relieves anger, valuable in manic-depressive cases. Has a sedative action on the heart, assists in bringing down high blood pressure, relieves insomnia, relieves muscular spasms and pains. Useful for menstrual problems. Clears the spleen and the liver. Keeps insects at bay and makes an excellent repellant for snakes. Purifies the air. Promotes growth of new skin cells, great healing effect on burns and sunburn, acne, psoriasis, boils, fungal growths, and scarring. A helpful oil for headache preparations. All in all, lavender is the best essential oil to keep on hand, due to its usefulness and affordability. Blends well with bergamot, chamomile, citronella, lemon, and pine.

Lemon (Citrus limon): Fresh, sharp citrus aroma. It is antacid, antineuralgic, antirheumatic, antiseptic, astringent, bactericide, diuretic, emollient, insecticide, and laxative. Helps to clear thoughts. Tonic to the circulatory system. liquefies the blood and aids flow, thereby easing pressure on varicose veins. Used to bring down high blood pressure. Helpful for nosebleeds. Eases painful cold sores and herpes. May be helpful with constipation and cellulite. Relieves headaches and migraines. Soothes insect bites and stings. Blends well with chamomile, eucalyptus, lavender and rose.

Lemongrass (Cymbopogon citratus): Sweet and lemony aroma. It is antidepressant, antiseptic, bactericide, diuretic, fungicide and insecticide. Stimulates the mind, lifts the spirit. Stimulates appetite, helpful with colic and indigestion. Prevents spread of contagious diseases. Great for aching muscles. Relieves tired legs. Relieves fatigue and jet lag. Aids in the flow of milk in nursing mothers. Blends well with cedarwood, basil, lavender, neroli, niaouli and tea tree.

Lime (Citrus auranttifolia): Restorative. Very stimulating in cases of apathy, depression and anxiety. Eases coughs and chest congestion. Encourages appetite, may assist in anorexia. Assists in treating alcoholism because of its disinfecting and restorative properties. Blends well with bergamot, geranium, lavender, rose and ylang ylang.

Mandarin (Citrus, reticulata): Citrus scent. Calming, soothing agent, astringent, skin conditioner. Blends well with basil, bergamot, chamomile, clary sage, geranium, grapefruit, lavender, lemon lime, neroli, orange, rose.

Marjoram, Spanish (Origanum margorana): Warm, penetrating and slightly spicy aroma. It is analgesic, antiseptic, antispasmodic, digestive, expectorant, sedative, and laxativeVery effective in dealing with painful muscles, mostly in the lower back area. Assists with swollen joints, good as after-sports rub. Seems to lower high blood pressure. Soothes digestion, may help with stomach cramps, constipation and flatulence. May be effective against seasickness. Alleviates stuffed-up feeling during colds. May be useful in relieving painful periods. Blends well with bergamot, cedarwood, orange, and rosewood.

Melissa (Melissa officinalis): (Sweet Balm, Lemon Balm) Distilled from lemon balm, this is true Melissa. It takes approximately 1.5 tons of the plant to obtain a pound of true Melissa essential oil, thus the expensive price of this true essential oil. This oil has proved useful in: oily skin, acne, cold sores, herpes, fungal infections, chronic coughs, colds (with headache), slowing rapid breathing, lowering blood pressure, colic, nausea, indigestion, menstrual pain & problems, regulating menstrual cycle, anxiety, depression, insomnia, migraine, tension, anger.

Myrrh (Commiphora myrrha): Smoky and slightly musky aroma. It is antiseptic, astringent, deodorant, disinfectant and diuretic. Best avoided during pregnancy as it is an emmenagogue. Seems to lift feelings of weakness, apathy and lack of incentive. Also has a cooling effect on heated emotions. Due to its drying action is effective against excessive mucous in the lungs. Recommended using in cases of bronchitis, colds, sore throats, and coughs. Excellent for mouth and gum disorders; it is the best treatment for mouth ulcers, gingivitis and bleeding or spongy gums. Eases flatulence and hemorrhoids. Stimulates and invigorates the immune system. Of great benefit in cases of scanty periods, leucorrhea and clearing obstructions in the womb. Blends well with clove frankincense, lavender and sandalwood.

Myrtle (Myrtus communis): Fresh, slightly sweet and penetrating. Antiseptic, astringent, bactericide, and expectorant. May soothe feelings of anger. Particularly useful with pulmonary disorders especially when accompanied by night sweats. Combats excessive moisture and clears sinusitis. Eases hemorrhoids and diarrhea. Could stem leucorrhea, said to be an effective tonic to the womb. Keeps vermin away. Could be useful in treatment of acne as well as clearing blemishes and bruises. May also alleviate the scaling appearance of psoriasis. Blends well with coriander, lavender, rosemary and tea tree.

Neroli (Citrus aurantium): Beautiful floral fragrance. It is antidepressant, antiseptic, antispasmodic, aphrodisiac, deodorant, digestive and sedative. Very relaxing, rather hypnotic, relieves chronic anxiety, depression and stress. Good in cases of insomnia. Assists with nerve pain, headaches and vertigo. Due to its calming effect may be beneficial to sexual problems and said to be an effective aphrodisiac. May relieve menopausal symptoms of irritability and tearfulness. Due to its antispasmodic action, it calms the intestines and is helpful with colitis and diarrhea. Blends well with bergamot, geranium, jasmine, lavender, lime, rose and ylang ylang.

Niaouli (Melaleuca virdiflora): Slightly sweet, penetrating aroma. It is analgesic, antiseptic, bactericide, insecticide and decongestant. Clears the head and may aid in concentration. Helps to fight infection by increasing white blood cell and antibody activity. Due to its pain relieving properties, may be of aid in rheumatism and neuralgia. Blends well with coriander, fennel, juniper, orange and peppermint.

Nutmeg (Myristica fragrans): Spicy, warm and nutty odor, clear oil. Considered analgesic and neurotonic. Indicated for extreme tiredness and used in massage blends for aching joints. Inhaled can cause nausea. One drop of Nutmeg with 20-40 drops of Orange is wonderful for the home. Blends well with citrus oils.

Orange, Sweet (Citrus aurantium) Zesty, refreshing citrus fragrance. It is antidepressant, antiseptic, antispasmodic, digestive and sedative. Prolonged use and high dosage may irritate sensitive skin and there's a chance of phototoxicity on skin exposed to the sun. Relieves gloomy thoughts and depression. Dispels stress. Revives one when bored. Calms the stomach in nervous states, assists with diarrhea and constipation. May encourage appetite; don't use if dieting. Very good for painful and sore muscles. Has a possibility of bringing down high level of cholesterol in the blood. Blends well with cinnamon, coriander, clove, frankincense, jasmine, lavender and rose.

Oregano (Origanum vulgare): Analgesic, antirheumatic, antispasmodic, antiseptic, disinfectant, emmenagogue, expectorant, laxative, antibiotic, and stomachic. A very potent oil, could irritate the mucous membranes. Best avoided in pregnancy. It's main effect seems to be on the digestive system, soothing the stomach, liver and spleen. Calms intestinal spasms. May combat acidity, stomach gas, and encourage appetite. May alleviate symptoms of asthma and whooping cough. Has some effect on skin parasites. Blends well with basil, fennel, geranium and pine.

Palamarosa (Cymbopogon martini): bactericide, and febrifuge. Refreshes and clarifies the mind. May be effective in cases of fever by reducing temperature. Acts as a tonic to the digestive system. Stimulates the appetite, may be helpful in cases of anorexia nervosa. May ease stiff joints. Blends well with bergamot, citronella, jasmine, lavender, and rose.

Parsley Seed (Petroselinum sativum): Somewhat herby aroma with spicy undertones. It is antiseptic, antispasmodic, aphrodisiac, digestive, expectorant, emmenagogue, laxative and parturient. Some precautions to be taken with this very powerful oil: Care is needed with dosage, otherwise dizziness may result. Should not be used in pregnancy or during painful menstruation as it may induce contractions of the womb. Best avoided in cases of kidney disease and peptic ulcers. Debatable whether should be used in massage. It is a very strong diuretic, stimulates the kidneys and could effectively clear cystitis and urinary stones. Rather useful in childbirth since it stimulates contractions during labor. Could well promote flow of breast milk and seems to relieve hardening of the breasts. While having a calming action on the digestion, it also stimulates the appetite. Useful also for flatulence. Apparently, takes the sting out of insect bites. Clear wounds and bruises by stimulating the blood flow. Good for keeping head lice away. Blends well with lavender, lime and orange.

Patchouli (Pogostemon patchouli): A strong, earthy fragrance, sweet and spicy also. It is antidepressant, antiseptic, aphrodisiac, astringent, deodorant, fungicide and insecticide. May cause loss of appetite. Its odor may be little too persistent for some people. Due to its strong astringent and cicatrizing properties, may be helpful for loose skin, especially after dieting. Seems to curb appetite also. Excellent in cases of diarrhea. Its diuretic properties are useful in cases of water retention and cellulite. Well known to increase libido. Relieves effects from insect bites. It is known as a tissue regenerator which helps regrowth of skin cells and the forming of scar tissue. Heals rough, cracked skin. Blends well with black pepper, clary sage, frankincense, geranium, lavender and myrrh.

Pennyroyal (Micromeria fruticosa): This EO should be used with extreme caution.. It is a well known emmenagogue; do not use during pregnancy. Has some use in menstrual difficulties, often used to bring on menstruation. Can be diluted either in alcohol or vinegar as a rub to kill fleas. Many aromatherapists will not use this oil as it can cause a spontaneous miscarriage in women who do not know they are pregnant. Deadly if consumed internally-do not ingest as a means to terminate pregnancy. It blends well with cedarwood and peppermint.

Pepper, Black (Pioer nigrum): Sharp, spicy aroma. Its analgesic, antiseptic, antispasmodic, aphrodisiac, cardiac, detoxifier, digestive, diuretic, laxative and stomachic. Useful for muscular aches and pains and muscular stiffness as it assists with dilation of local blood vessels. Good to use before excessive exertion. Assists with rheumatoid arthritis and temporary limb paralysis. Stimulates appetite. Expels wind, quells vomiting. Banishes excess fat, possibly by aiding digestion of protein; generally expels toxins. May be helpful with anemia as it aids the formation of new blood cells. Can bring down high temperatures. Blends well with basil, bergamot, cypress, grapefruit, lemon, and sandalwood.

Peppermint (Mentha piperita): Sharp, menthol fragrance. Analgesic, anesthetic, antispasmodic, astringent, decongestant, emmenagogue, expectorant, insecticide and stimulant. Should be kept away from eyes, likely to irritate skin and mucous membranes. Best avoided by pregnant women and nursing mothers as it may discourage flow of milk. May antidote homeopathic remedies. Said to relieve states of anger, hysteria and nervous trembling, excellent for mental fatigue and depression. On the body, it has a dual action: cooling when hot and warming when cold. As a remedy for colds, it halts mucous and fevers and encourages perspiration. Extremely important for its effect on the digestive system. Good for travel sickness, vomiting, diarrhea, constipation, colic and nausea.. Its cooling and pain relieving action seems to ease headaches, migraines and toothaches. Blends well with cedarwood, cypress, lavender, neroli and pine.

Petitgrain (Citrus bigarade): Has a fragrance that is alternately woody and floral. It is antidepressant, antispasmodic and deodorant. Calms anger and panic, refreshes the mind. Eases breathing and relaxes muscle spasms. Helpful with painful digestion by calming stomach muscles. Could help in clearing up skin blemishes and pimples. Blends well with bergamot, cedarwood, lavender, neroli, orange, rosewood and sandalwood.

Pine (Pinus sylvestris): Fresh, forest aroma. It is antiseptic, decongestant, deodorant, diuretic, expectorant, and sudorific. Known to refresh a tired mind and mental fatigue. It is a powerful antiseptic and helpful in cases of bronchitis, laryngitis and influenza. Has good effect on respiratory problems. Effective with cystitis and prostate problems and known as a general kidney cleanser. Its warming properties may relieve rheumatism, gout and arthritis. Reputedly effective on male sexual problems, possibly impotence. Blends well with cedarwood, clove, and niaouli.

Rose Otto (Rosa centifolia): Deep, sweet and flowery, an exquisite perfume. Also known as Damask Rose from Bulgaria. It is antidepressant, antiseptic, antispasmodic, aphrodisiac, bactericide, diuretic, emmenagogue, laxative, sedative. Since it is an emmenagogue, it is best avoided in pregnancy. Has a soothing effect on the emotions, particularly depression, grief, jealousy and resentment. Lifts and heart and eases nervous tension and stress. Calms PMS, promotes vaginal secretions and regulates the menstrual cycle. Helpful with sexual difficulties, particularly frigidity and impotence. Release the "happy" hormone dopamine. Activates sluggish blood circulation, relieving cardiac congestion and toning the capillaries. Relieves nausea, vomiting and constipation to some extent. Has a purging action on toxins, the Romans valued it for hangovers. Has a soothing action on sore throats and eases coughs. Useful for all skin types, though particularly good for mature, dry, hard or sensitive skin. Valuable treatment for broken thread veins. Blends well with bergamot, chamomile, clary sage, geranium, lavender, orange and sandalwood.

Rosemary (Rosamarinus officnalis): A refreshing herbal fragrance. It is analgesic, antidepressant, antirheumatic, antiseptic, antispasmodic, astringent, cicatrizing, digestive, diuretic, hypertensive and stomachache. Not suitable for people with epilepsy or high blood pressure. Avoid in pregnancy since it is an emmenagogue. Clears the head and aids memory. Clears headaches and migraines, especially when connected to gastric problems. May assist with vertigo. Helps to tone temporarily paralyzed limbs. Helps ease gout and tired, overworked muscles. Normalizes blood pressure. Could ease colitis, flatulence and stomach pains. Its diuretic properties may be useful with water retention during menstruation and may be effective with cellulite and obesity. Blends well with grapefruit, orange and peppermint.

Rosewood (Bois de Rose)(Aniba rosaeodora): Sweet, woody, floral and slightly spicy aroma. It is analgesic, antidepressant, antiseptic, aphrodisiac, deodorant, and insecticide. It is said to stabilize the central nervous system and could therefore have an overall balancing effect. Its acclaimed aphrodisiac properties may work wonders in restoring libido and could have some effect on sexual problems such as impotence and frigidity. Reputedly helpful for persons who have suffered sexual abuse. May relieve headaches when accompanied by nausea and may also relieve jet lag. Its deodorizing action helps the body cope with excess heat and moisture. Also valuable as an insect repellent.

Sage(Saliva officinalis): Soothing agent, energizing, stimulating. Blends well with rosemary and citrus oils. Useful for congestion, cough, and a traditional herb for space clearing in Native American traditions. Can be used to regulate menses.

Sandalwood (Santalum album): Woody, sweet and exotic aroma. Antiseptic, antispasmodic, aphrodisiac, astringent, diuretic, expectorant and sedative. Its lingering aroma often persists in clothing after washing. Avoid in states of depression as it may lower the mood even further. Its aphrodisiac properties are well known. Alleviates cystitis (massage in the kidney region where it has a purifying and anti-inflammatory action). Its aphrodisiac properties can relieve sexual problems such as frigidity, impotence, and was traditionally once was used to alleviate sexually transmitted diseases. Helpful with chest infections and sore throats. Aids sleep during colds and flu. Stimulates the immune system and keeps infection at bay. A spiritual oil used in mediation and prayer by many cultures. Particularly good for dry eczema as well as ageing and dehydrated skins. Relieves itching and inflammation. Blends well with frankincense, geranium, lavender, lemon, neroli, rose, and vetiver.

Spearmint (Mehtha spicata): Antispasmodic, emmenagogue, insecticide, and stimulant. Possibility of eye irritation, as well as sensitive skin. Avoid in pregnancy. Stimulates a tired mind. Helpful with digestive problems such as vomiting , flatulence, constipation and diarrhea. Seems to elieve hiccups and nausea. May help with seasickness. Releases retention of urine and dissolves kidney stones. It controls overabundance of breast milk. By the same token, it could stem the flow of heavy periods. It is said to ease labor. Good for headaches. May help sores and scabs. Blends well with basil, grapefruit and rosemary.

Spruce (Picea mariana): Fresh pine, bitter orange aroma. Recommended for relief of stress and anxiety. Also recommended for muscle aches and pains, aching joints, poor circulation, muscle spasms. It is been known to be helpful for bronchitis or asthma. Blends well with Lavender and Clary sage.

Tagetes (Tagetes minuta/glandulifera) A wild, sweet, fruity almost citrus-like smell. The therapeutic properties of Tagetes are anti-infectious, anti-microbial, antibiotic, anti-spasmodic, anti-parasitic, antiseptic, insecticide and sedative. Tagetes is a very powerful oil and should be used sparingly and should be avoided during pregnancy. The therapeutic properties of Tagetes are anti-infectious, anti-microbial, antibiotic, anti-spasmodic, anti-parasitic, antiseptic, insecticide and sedative. Tagetes is valuable in keeping insects at bay, and can help with parasitic and fungal infestation. It is used for chest infections, dilating the bronchi, facilitating the flow of mucus and dislodging congestion and can be used in cases of skin infections. It has a healing effect on wounds, cuts, calluses, blisters, and bunions. Tagetes can be useful for treating the respiratory system, infections of the skin and as an insect repellent.

Tangerine (Citrus tangelo): Sweet and tangy aroma. It is antiseptic, antispasmodic, sedative and stomachic. Could be phototoxic; care should be taken not to expose the skin to strong sunlight after treatment. Has an almost hypnotic effect on the mind. May be helpful with stress and tension due to its soothing action on the nervous system. Assists with gastric complaints, such as flatulence, diarrhea and constipation. Stimulates flow of bile which helps to digest fats. Assists with tired and aching limbs since it is a tonic to the vascular system. Could help smooth out stretch marks, particularly when blended with lavender and neroli. Blends well with basil, bergamot, chamomile, clary sage, frankincense, neroli, orange and rose.

Tea Tree (Melaleuca alternifolia): Fresh and sanitary, rather pungent aroma. Like lavender, it would take pages to list all the redeeming qualities of this oil. It is antibiotic, antiseptic, antiviral, bactericide, cicatrizing, expectorant, fungicide, insecticide and sedative. May cause irritation on sensitive areas of skin; however, along with Lavender, it is just about the only oil that is recommended to be used "neat" or straight from the bottle without dilution. Its most important usage is to help the immune system fight off infectious diseases. Sweats toxins out of the body. Indicated for influenza, cold sores, and gingivitis. A series of massage with this oil before surgery will help to fortify the body. Its strong antiviral and germicidal properties are useful in repeated infections. Its fungicidal properties help clear vaginal thrush and is of value with genital infections generally. Alleviates urinary tract problems such as cystitis. Gives relief to genital and anal itching as well as general itching from chicken pox to rashes caused by insect bites. Said to give some protection against x-ray therapy in breast cancer. It will apparently reduce scarring when applied before treatment, as the protective film will guard against very deep penetration of the x-rays. Reduces pus in infected wounds. Useful with burns, sores, sunburn, ringworm, warts, herpes and athletes foot. Helpful with dry conditions of the scalp as well as dandruff. Blends well with cinnamon, clove, cypress, eucalyptus, ginger, lavender, and thyme.

Thyme (Thymus vulgaris): A rather sweet and strongly herbal fragrance. It is well known as being antirheumatic, antiseptic, antispasmodic, aphrodisiac, cardiac, cicatrizing, diuretic, emmenagogue, expectorant, and insecticide. This is a very potent oil, one of the strongest antiseptics and toxicity is possible with prolonged use. Not to be used in cases of high blood pressure nor in pregnancy. Activates brain cells, thereby aiding memory and concentration. Has been used in massage for those suffering for MS with proven results. Helps the body fight disease. May be recommended for rheumatism, gout and arthritis. May stop nosebleeds. Helps with sluggish digestion and wind. Speeds delivery in childbirth and expelling the afterbirth. A tonic for the scalp and may be effective with dandruff and hair loss. Blends well with bergamot, cedarwood, chamomile, and lemon.

(Lemon)Verbena (Lippia citriodora): Smells of sweet lemons. It is antiseptic, antispasmodic, aphrodisiac, digestive, emollient, insecticide and stomachic. Recent pharmacological tests have proven this oil to be phototoxic and a strong skin sensitizer. Not recommended for massages. It is famous for banishing depression due to its tonic, soothing effect on the parasympathetic nervous system. Works on the digestive system, especially controlling stomach spasms and cramps, nausea, indigestion and flatulence. Keeps down skin puffiness. Blends well with basil, bergamot, chamomile, geranium, neroli, rose, and rosemary.

Vetivert (Vetiveria zizanoides): Deep, smoky, earthy aroma. It is antiseptic, aphrodisiac, sedative, nervine. It is a calming oil, excellent for stress and tension. Settles the nerves. May be useful in helping people ease off tranquilizers. Said to cleanse the aura (the energy field around the body) and to strengthen the auric shield which can be instrumental in keeping out disease. A tonic to the reproductive system and its relaxing quality seems to have some effect on tension underlying sexual problems. Blends well with frankincense, geranium, grapefruit, jasmine, lavender, rose, sandalwood and ylang ylang.

Wintergreen (Gaultheria procumbens): Very refreshing aroma. Use with caution, the EO is approximately 99% salicylate, the main ingredient in aspirin (irritant, sensitizing). Use tiny amounts in muscle/joint blends, patch test. Not recommended for usage in persons who take aspirin regularly.

Yarrow (Achillea millifoleum): Common name is Milfoil (Achillea millefolium). Its aroma is dry and herbaceous with pale yellow to brilliant blue color. It's a well-known anti-inflammatory and is indicated for prostate or menstrual problems and neuralgia. Because of its high content of Azulene, Yarrow oil is used in skin care for acne, eczema and inflammation to minimize varicose veins and reduce scars. Yarrow provides protection from ticks. It is also used to counter radiation.

Ylang Ylang (Canagana odorata): Sweet, floral, heavy aroma. Ylang Ylang both relaxes and arouses; in Europe, therapists use it for sexual dysfunction. It is antidepressant, antiseptic, aphrodisiac,sedative. Excessive use may lead to headaches and nausea. Could possibly irritate sensitive skins and indicated against use on inflammatory skin conditions and dermatitis. Could ease feelings of anger, anxiety, shock, panic and fear.. Has a tonic and stimulating effect on the scalp promoting a more luxurious hair growth. Blends well with bergamot, citronella, jasmine, lavender, lemon, rose, sandalwood and verbena.

Using Aromatherapy With Other Holistic Modalities

Essential oils go together with all different kinds of healing modalities. They can be used with Crystal Therapy, oils placed on the stones and then the stones placed on the body. Reflexology, oils diluted in a carrier oil for a refreshing foot or hand massage. Acupressure, Massage. Put some oil in a diffuser during a Reiki session. Oils can be used to set moods and for medicinal uses. Experiment! play with your oils to see what you can come up with. Remember a little goes a long way.

Zodiac Oils

Capricorn- Rosemary
Aquarius- Frankincense
Pisces- Bergamot
Aries- Lavender
Taurus- Patchouli
Gemini- Chamomile
Cancer- Basil
Leo- Vetivert
Virgo- Rose
Libra- Clary Sage
Scorpio- Sandalwood
Sagittarius- Juniper

Crafts and Projects

You can use dried herbs and flowers in combination with essential oils to make great little **sachets and potpourri**. To do, Place dried herb of choice in a brown paper bag, place a few drops of essential oil (s) in bag, shake well or blend with hands, close bag and leave overnight. Put in a bowl or cloth. To refresh put back in a bag and shake well, this releases the oils once again for a fresh scent. Or tie the herbs up in a piece of felt for drawer sachets.

Aromatherapy candles: get some melt n' pour wax, melt down, let cool a bit and add oils. Remember to let wax cool or it will evaporate the oil. Pour into molds or any container or jar, add a wick, and let cool and enjoy. You can make tarts the same way, just omit the wick and pour in shallow molds.

You can keep a blotter in a **locket** around my neck, can change scent according to your mood or what I do is keep adding to it. I can't even describe how good it smells.

Lip balms and glosses are easy to make- some cocoa butter, sweet almond oil and a few drops of your favorite oil for gloss, add a little beeswax for balms.

A good one for Christmas is cocoamint lip balm- 1.5oz cocoa butter, 1 oz beeswax, 1.5 oz shea butter, 2 capsules vitamin E, 10-15 drops Peppermint oil. Put in tubes or containers. Add a few drops of sent to a good **lotion** and you wont keep it around long.

Bath salts are easy- 1 ½ cups Epsom salt, 1c baking soda, 1/2 c salt 1/8 or less oils. Or just sea salt and oil.

Bath bombs- 1-2 parts Epsom salt, 2 parts baking soda, 1 part cornstarch,1-2 parts citric acid, 1 part grapeseed oil, kneed till dough like (not sticky) add drops of oil till you like the scent, roll into balls and wrap in cellophane till ready to use.

Soap- glycerin chunks melt in the microwave and you stir in oils last minute as you pour into molds. This is a project that takes minutes that is fun for children and holiday gift making.

Reflexology

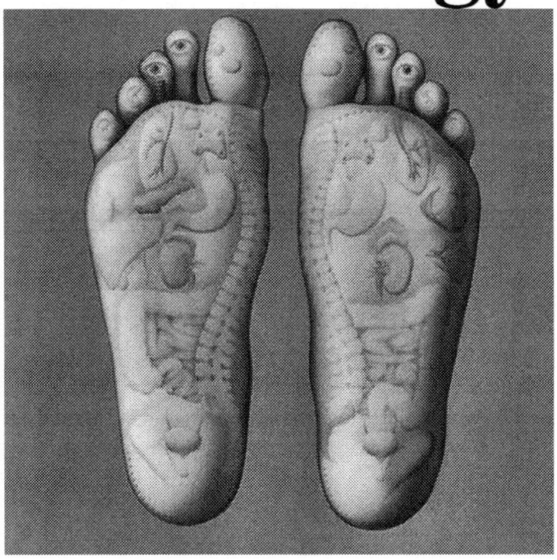

What is Reflexology?

Reflexology is the application of pressure and movement to the feet to effect corresponding parts of the body. Reflexologists know that the feet are a mirror image of the body. By applying one of several techniques and grips, a reflexologist can break up patterns of stress in other parts of the body.

Reflexology is an art and science that goes well beyond foot massage. It is based on psychological and neurological studies. There are specific pressure points targeted in reflexology. These points correspond with all body parts, meaning that each body organ has a specific place on the foot to be manipulated in order to stimulate well-being.

How Does Reflexology Work?

There are many theories but in our approach we look at the nervous system as the explanation of reflexology's working. Pressure applied to the feet generates a signal through the peripheral nervous system. From there it enters the central nervous system where it is processed in various parts of the brain. It is then relayed to the internal organs to allocate the necessary adjustments in fuel and oxygen. Finally a response is fashioned that is sent onto the motor system.

This message is fed forward to adjust the body's tone or overall tension level. If applied properly the tone will reset itself to a lower operating tempo. A lower operating tempo means a lessening of stress and less wear and tear on the body's systems.

The Chinese discovered that this energy or Chi circulates along 12 meridians that are pathways in the body. Reflexology opens the energy pathway, energizing the physical and mental aspects of the client. When reflexes in the feet are stimulated an involuntary response is touched in organs and glands connected by pathways to these specific reflexes. A consistent reaction is set, causing psychological changes to occur and a reduction in stress, which causes approximately 70% of all disorders.

History

Reflexology began in China about 5000 years ago. Drawings on walls in Egyptian caves depict pressure therapy was performed on the feet and hands. In 1913, William Fitzgerald, M.D. (a.k.a. The Father of Modern Reflexology) found that the application of pressure to various parts of the body removed pain in other areas, and thus reduced the need for anesthesia in surgery and other procedures. In the 1930s, Eunice Ingham, a nurse, established herself as a pioneer in the field of reflexology when she discovered that in using a pressure technique across the soles of the feet, she was able to stimulate and heal other parts of the body, rather than to merely numb sensations of pain. In recent years, there has been a resurgence of interest in hands-on healing techniques such as reflexology as people become disenchanted with or cannot afford the costly surgery- and/or drug-based methods common to traditional Western medicine. Simply put, what people today are rediscovering is that Nature has always provided us with the means by which to heal us and maintain good health.

The Anatomy of the Foot

The human foot combines mechanical complexity and structural strength. The ankle serves as foundation, shock absorber, and propulsion engine. The foot can sustain enormous pressure (several tons over the course of a one-mile run) and provides flexibility and resiliency. The average foot contains 26 small bones: 2 sesamoids (smaller bones), 114 ligaments, and 20 muscles. They are joined together by connective tissue, blood vessels, and nerves, then covered in layers of skin. There are 33 joints and more than 100 muscles, tendons and ligaments all balanced on 2 arches. In each foot there are 14 toe bones and 3 phalanges in each toe except the big toe only having 2.

These components work together to provide the body with support, balance, and mobility. A structural flaw or malfunction in any one part can result in the development of problems elsewhere in the body. Conversely, abnormalities in other parts of the body can lead to problems in the feet. This is why it is very important to wear appropriate fitting shoes.

The forefoot is composed of the five toes (called phalanges) and their connecting long bones (metatarsals). Each toe (phalanx) is made up of several small bones. The big toe (hallux) has two phalanges, two joints (interphalangeal joints), and two tiny, round sesamoid bones that enable it to move up and down. The other four toes each have three bones and two joints. The phalanges are connected to the metatarsals by five metatarsal phalange joints at the ball of the foot. The forefoot bears half the body's weight and balances pressure on the ball of the foot.

The midfoot has five irregularly shaped tarsal bones, which form the foot's arch, and serves as a shock absorber. The bones of the midfoot are connected to the forefoot and the hindfoot by muscles and the plantar fascia (arch ligament).

The hindfoot is composed of three joints and links the midfoot to the ankle (talus). The top of the talus is connected to the two long bones of the lower leg (tibia and fibula), forming a hinge that allows the foot to move up and down. The heel bone (calcaneus) is the largest bone in the foot. It joins the talus to form the subtalar joint, which enables the foot to rotate at the ankle. A layer of fat cushions the bottom of the heel bone.

There are 20 muscles in the foot that give the foot its shape by holding the bones in position and expand and contract to impart movement.

The Main Muscles of the Foot

The anterior tibial, which enables the foot to move upward;
The posterior tibiae, which supports the arch;
The peroneal tibiae, which controls movement on the outside of the ankle;
The extensors, which help the ankle raise the toes to step forward;
The flexors, which help stabilize the toes against the ground.
Smaller muscles enable the toes to lift and curl.

There are elastic tissues (tendons) in the foot that connect the muscles to the bones and joints. The largest and strongest tendon of the foot is the Achilles tendon, which extends from the calf muscle to the heel. Its strength and joint function facilitate running, jumping, walking up stairs, and raising the body onto the toes.

Ligaments hold the tendons in place and stabilize the joints. The longest of these, the plantar fascia, forms the arch on the sole of the foot from the heel to the toes. By stretching and contracting, it allows the arch to curve or flatten, providing balance and giving the foot strength to initiate the act of walking. Medial ligaments on the inside and lateral ligaments on outside of the foot provide stability and enable the foot to move up and down.

Skin, blood vessels, and nerves give the foot its shape and durability and provide cell regeneration, essential muscular nourishment, and control its varied movements.

Side View of Foot Bones

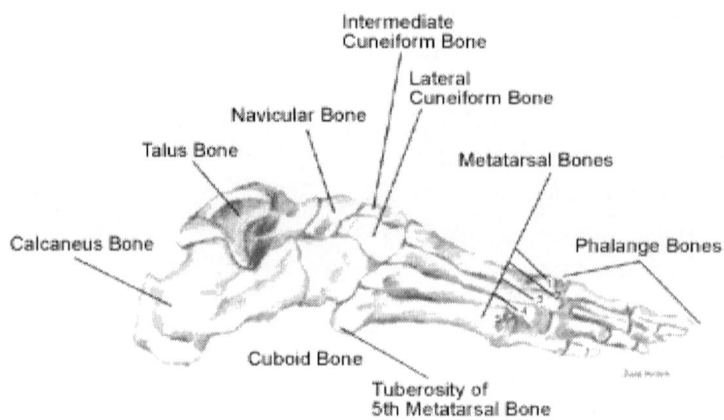

Top View of Foot Bones

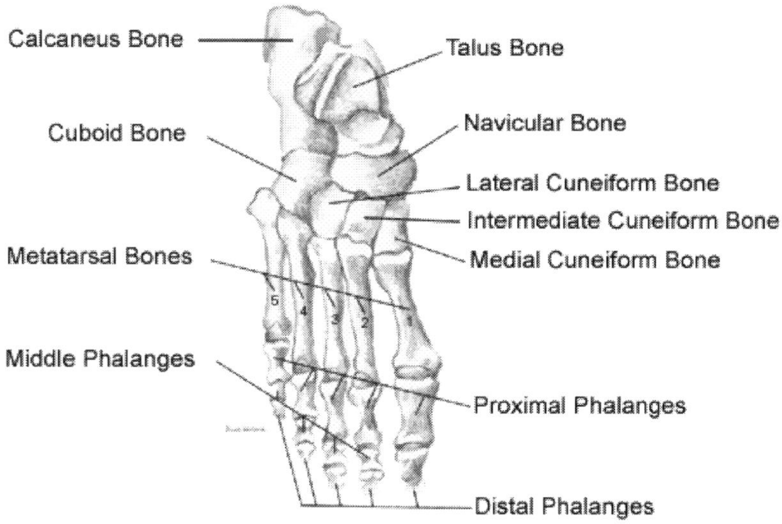

Foot Care

Taking care of your feet not only keeps them looking good but also has health benefits. Good hygiene is import. Washing the feet daily to remove dead skin cells helps the foot breathe. The foot loses about a 1/4 cup of moisture a day. This causes the foot to become moist and soggy, making it easier for bacteria, blisters, fungi, and bromhidrosis (smelly feet) to form. Using creams and oils to keep the condition of the skin soft and supple and Pedicures are beneficial. Pumice stones are wonderful for taking off dry rough spots. Footbaths in herbs or oils are one of my favorite treatments.

Holistic Approach

70% of the population lives with too much strain, worry and tension. Reflexology can be of great assistance to those under constant stress. Over a period of time an imbalance can occur to the bodily functions causing any number of illnesses. The blood and nerve supply to an organ or gland can be dramatically restricted. It is believed that working on the reflexes cause the body to eliminate unwanted toxins and pollutants from the body. Reflexology procedures aim directly to correct physical and emotional imbalance within the body. The energy pathways are opened up when the reflexologist correctly stimulates the reflexes on the feet. The body's immune system can be boosted. Energy can be revitalized and one's whole system rebalanced without the need of drugs.

Insomnia sufferers find treatments encourage deep quality sleep and give most people a sense of deep relaxation and profound peace. Athletes who have regular reflexology sessions have fewer injuries. Reflexology treatment aids the delivery of blood to such needed areas. Post-operative patients receiving reflexology treatments on average stay in the hospital three to five days less than those who do not. Reflexology can benefit: arthritis, asthma, emphysema, hay fever, constipation, and incontinence, digestive disorders, hernia, ulcers, gall stones, infertility, impotence and prostate problems, heart and circulatory diseases, migraine headaches, all disorders of the sense organs, throat neck and back pain; hormonal and menopausal conditions. As you can see, reflexology can help almost any condition.

Meridians

Meridian is a general term for the channels and their collaterals. Jing (channels) in Chinese means "route". Each meridian is predominantly either Yin or Yang. Yin meridians flow upwards. Yang meridians flow downwards. Yin meridians are associated with the Zang organ while yang meridians are associated with the Fu organs. So each major meridian gets its name by the organ with which it is associated:

1 **Lung Meridian**: its starting point is on the middle of the stomach. It runs through the outside of the chest, then turns down from the collarbone into the inside of the arm and ends on the top of the thumb. The Lung meridian is usually seen as the starting point in the cycle of Qi. There are 11 acupuncture points lying along the course of the meridian. Associated Symptoms: cough, asthma, tightness in chest, pain in the top of the shoulder or the inside of the arm.

2 **Large Intestine Meridian:** the first point is on the inside of the top section of the index finger. It runs up, outside the arm and turns in towards the clavicle into the lower jawbone, and ends via the corner of the mouth closed to the nose. There are 20 points along this meridian. Associated Symptoms: nosebleed, sore throat, toothache, stiffness of the shoulder, pain of the outside of the arm, and abdominal pain.

3 **Stomach Meridian:** It begins at the side of the nose, runs along the lower jaw to the vicinity of the chest and stomach, then passes the navel and goes down along the front of the leg. It ends on the top part of the second toe. 45 points lie along this meridian. Associated Symptoms: fever, nosebleed, chest pain, cramps in the legs, loss of appetite, distension of the abdomen, diarrhea.

4 **Spleen Meridian:** It starts from the outside of the big toe, runs up along the inside of the leg, passes the abdomen, and ends below the armpit. There are 21 points along this meridian. Associated Symptoms: upper abdominal pain, jaundice or diarrhea, vomiting, tongues stiffness, painful or swollen knees.

5 **Heart Meridian**: the starting point is located beneath the chest. Through the armpit, it runs along the inside of the arm and ends on the top of the little finger. This meridian links only 9 points. Associated Symptoms: fever, pain in the chest, palpitations, cold sweats, feeling of thirst, pain of the inside of the shoulder.

6 **Small Intestine Meridian:** It begins on the top of the little finger, runs on the outside of the forearm, crosses the shoulder joint and jawbone, and ends at the outer corner of the ear. There are 19 points on this course. Associated Symptoms: ringing in the ears, sore throat, and pain in the outside of the shoulder.

7 **Urinary/Bladder Meridian:** starts at the inner corner of the eye and runs across the top of the head. At the neck it divides into two branches that run down the back in parallel. One reaches the heel through the leg and ends on the little toe. The other ends in the hollow of the knee. This meridian touches 67 points. Associated Symptoms: nasal congestion, watering eyes, or other nose and eye problems, headaches, bed-wetting, pain in the outside of the legs, etc.

8 **Kidney Meridian:** The starting point is on the front part of the little toe. Across the center of the foot bottom, it runs along the inside of the leg and then up the abdomen, and ends on the ends of the collarbone. The meridian comprises 27 points. Associated Symptoms: hyperactivity, asthma, coughing of blood, sore throat, blurring of vision, ringing in the ears, tiredness, loss of sex drive, etc.

9 **Pericardium Meridian:** its starting point lies at the center of the chest. It runs across the armpit and along the inside of the arm, and ends on the top of the index finger. There are only 9 points along the course. Associated Symptoms: chest pain, palpitations, anxiety, mental disturbance, and stiffness of the arms.

10 **Sanjiao Meridian:** it begins at the ring finger, up the outside of the arm, across the shoulder and neck, and around the ear where it ends on the side of the eye. A total 23 points lie on this meridian. Associated Symptoms: hearing problems, sore throat, pain in the arm, abdominal pain, and urine retention.

11 **Gall Bladder Meridian:** Beginning at the outer corner of the eye, it runs across the temple and beside the ear, past the shoulder joint into the side of the body and along the outside of the leg to the end of the fourth toe. There are 44 points along this

course. Associated Symptoms: headache, chest or upper abdominal pain, and stiffness of legs, dizziness.

12 **Liver Meridian**: It starts at the big toe, crosses the top of the foot, runs along the inside of the leg, past the bladder, and ends at the stomach. It consists of 14 points along the meridian. Associated Symptoms: swollen lower abdomen, feeling of tightness in the stomach, vomiting, etc. The liver meridian completes the circulation of Qi that starts in the heart meridian, and passes it on to the heart meridian again.

When to Perform Reflexology

Reflexology can be done anytime and anywhere. Consistency is the key. The results from China seem to be that they do reflexology once a day for six days in two week segments. Then they review the results and do more segments as necessary. This requires self-help and family help as well as the guidance of practitioners. The practitioner can give you a quality signal to break up the pattern of stress but you and your family can provide the quantity to help break it up. Build reflexology into your life. It is easy to do reflexology while doing other activities. Put a foot roller under your desk or work your hands while waiting for the kids at school.

What to Expect from a Session

Reflexology sessions in general last from 30 minutes to an hour. It is a clothed session with only the removal of shoes and socks as a requirement. The reflexologist will use a chair or a table. Some use lotion or oil. However, dry technique is common. Reflexologists use pressure, stretch, and movement to work through the foot methodically. The whole foot should be worked in most circumstances. Both feet should be covered as well. The reflexologist should work within your comfort zone. Too much pressure can actually be harmful and could lead to injury. But personal preference is something you should communicate with your reflexologist.

Do not rely on a reflexologist for medical help, nor should a reflexologist allow a client to view them as a medical doctor. The reflexologist is limited to complementing medicine, not replacing it.

You should feel relaxed at the end of a session. How long that relaxation lasts is a good indicator of the effectiveness of the session. Tell your reflexologist your response to the session during your follow up. This is very helpful information.

Finally, enjoy the session. Be careful that talking doesn't interfere with the relaxation effect. Discussing world politics is probably something best left to another time.

Sessions

Before a session, you should ground and center yourself. You should be in the right mind to promote healing. You can do this by deep breathing or meditating. There are many ways to center yourself; you have to find the right way for you. The environment should be relaxing, so the client can relax. Leading the client through deep breathing or a meditation is a great way to start and end the session. Before the session it helps the client to relax to promote healing. After the session it relaxes the client to help maintain the energy that you have balanced.

Before working on anybody, you should give them an intake form to fill out to find what needs worked on, if they have any contraindications. It is a good idea keep track of the points that you have used during a session and if they worked or not. It is also good to ask your client each time what has improved and what hasn't and keep a record on that information.

When working on points, start out with light pressure and then gradually go deeper. When you are done working on a point, gradually lift your hand. This helps with the circulation. You should apply enough firm pressure so that the client feels it qualifies as "deep" but not enough so that your client is in pain. You should hold a point one minute or so to relax the point. You can stay as long as five minutes on a point that is really giving them trouble, but no more than that will offer any greater benefit. To stimulate any point, however, you need to hold the point four to five seconds at a time minimum, with 30 seconds to one minute being the standard time. Do not be abrupt, forceful, or work the points in a jarring way.

RIGHT FOOT

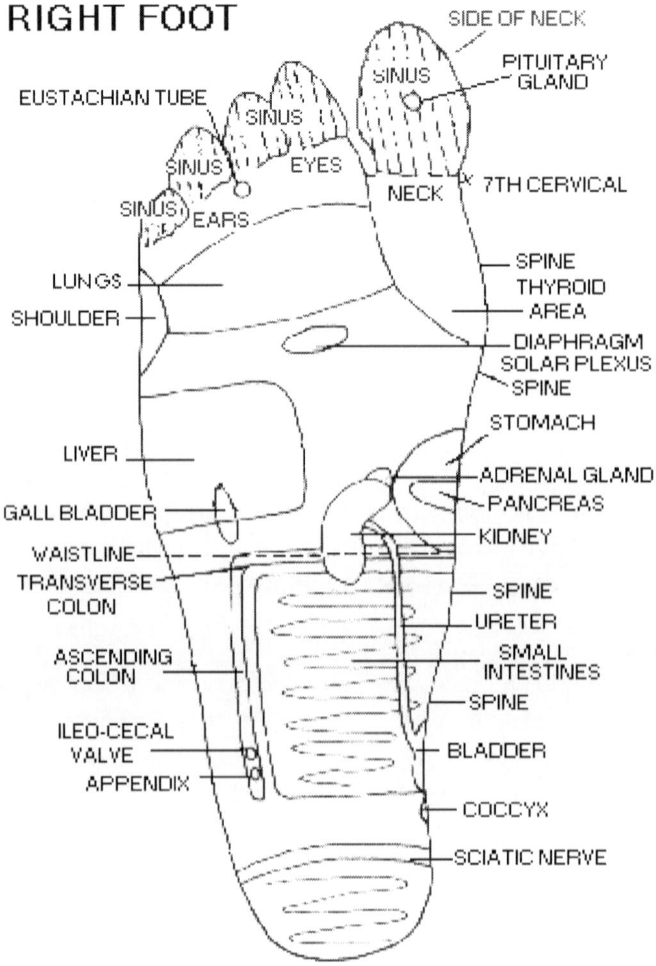
SIDE OF NECK
PITUITARY GLAND
EUSTACHIAN TUBE
SINUS
SINUS
SINUS
SINUS
EYES
EARS
NECK
7TH CERVICAL
SPINE
LUNGS
THYROID AREA
SHOULDER
DIAPHRAGM
SOLAR PLEXUS
SPINE
STOMACH
LIVER
ADRENAL GLAND
PANCREAS
GALL BLADDER
KIDNEY
WAISTLINE
TRANSVERSE COLON
SPINE
URETER
ASCENDING COLON
SMALL INTESTINES
SPINE
ILEO-CECAL VALVE
BLADDER
APPENDIX
COCCYX
SCIATIC NERVE

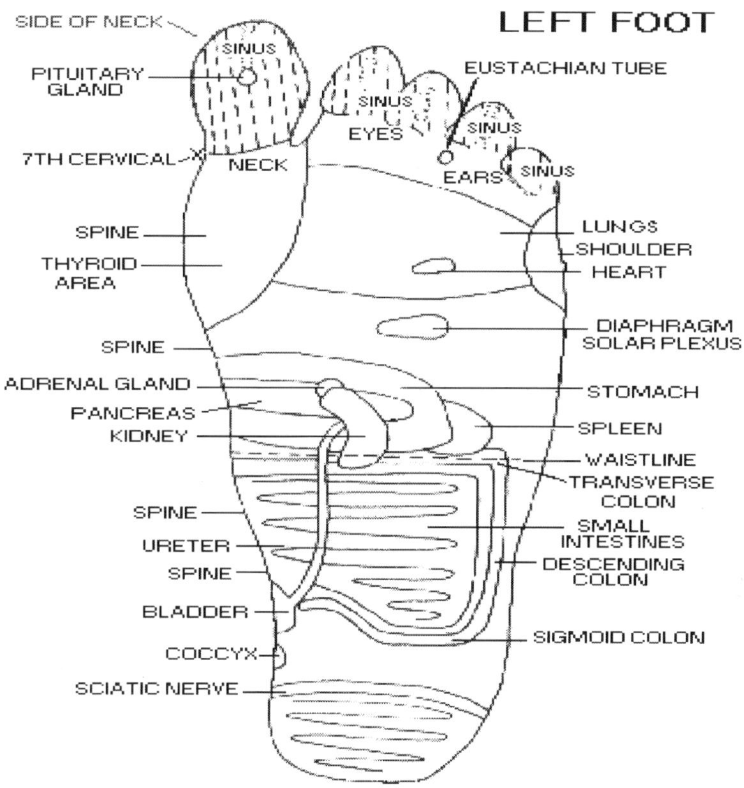

Technique and Preparation

In preparation for treatment, individuals should be informed of what Reflexology is and what you will be doing. The first thing to do with a client is to get their medical history. Also, ask if the client is currently taking a prescribed medication. If they are on pain medication, be careful not to work too deeply, as their pain responses are diminished. Caution the client that alcohol, tobacco, and recreational drugs will slow the benefits of alternative therapies and should not be used. Other drugs may affect the outcome of your therapy. If they are on any medications, please explain this with them. Your main objective after filling out the chart is to assess the clients best needs. Make the room comfortable, soft music may be played. Essential oils in a diffuser to relax the patient may be used. You will examine their feet, looking for any problem areas. Where these problem areas are will tell you where the source of disease is. Here this list will describe different disorders:

Bunions
Hammertoe
Calluses and Corns
Athlete's foot
Ingrown toenail
Thickened toenail
Fungal infection
Flat feet
Heal spur
Plantar warts
Eczema
Arthritis
Gout

Firmly massage the bottoms of the feet, but do not cause pain. Always start with the right foot, and massage UP the area corresponding to the Ascending Colon. Then finish the rest of the foot. When you are finished with the right foot, start on the left foot by massaging DOWN the Descending colon, then finish the rest of the foot. When massaging the foot, notice where there is pain. These areas of pain correspond to an organ that may be weak or dis-eased. Pay extra attention to this area by giving them extra massage time. A session takes 30-45 minutes.

Grips

How you hold the foot is important or pressure won't be right. Use one hand to support the foot, the other hand to apply pressure. Push in with your thumb-- pretend your thumb is moving inside of a square. Do not move your thumb off of the spot, but rotate it around the spot. The sequence for pressure is press in, rotate 3times, lift, then move onto the next spot.

Grip 1. Sinus, Bronchi, lungs heart, chronic eyes and ears
Left hand usually supports while the right is the worker.
The rotating thumb technique will put pressure on the reflex points while the fist clenched keeps the thumb free.

Grip 2. Pituitary gland, brain mater, eyes and ears
The support hand holds the foot close to the toes. With the other hand, place fingers on top of the foot pointing downward, the thumb positioned to work under the toes.

Grip 3. Pituitary Gland
If grip 2 isn't sufficient in finding the pituitary gland this is an alternative method.

Cup the foot with the support hand while useing the knuckle of the forefinger to rotate.

Grip 4. Upper Lymphatic
The left hand supports while the right works with the thumb to support. The fingers massage the top of the foot. Mainly use the middle finger. Reach down the foot as far as possible to rotate. When you get to the webs apply pressure. Repeat between each toe using the bones of the metatarsal as a guide.

Grip 5. Thyroid, parathyroid, neck
This reflex covers the whole ball of the foot, most importantly the half circle shape at the base of the bone. To hit this spot you must get the right angle to get up and under. Use the working hand thumb, and press and rotate at the half circle of the ball over the neck reflex to cover the section at the base of the big toe.

Grip 6. Liver, gall bladder, stomach, pancreas, spleen, intestines, kidneys, adrenals, uterus
To get this position right you must be able to swivel. Always work the outside with the left hand and support with the other hand. Rotating thumb technique is used.

Grip 7. Bladder uterus/prostate, ovaries, testes, spine, hip, elbow, shoulder.
Cup the foot in the palm of the working hand. This is mainly used when working the sides of the feet.

Grip 8. Solar Plexus
Gently grip the foot from the top until you see an indentation in the center of the foot. That is the Solar Plexus. Watch the client's breath for this one. When they inhale press in there, when they exhale release the pressure.

Session Relaxation Technique Description

1. Achilles tendon stretch- Cup hands so heel rests in palm. Grasp top of foot in the "Standard Support Grip" (SSG). Pull tops of foot towards you then back. Repeat 2-3 times on each foot.

2. Ankle rotation- Cup back of foot for support. With thumb on side of ankle grasp foot at the base of big toe in SSG rotate foot 260 8 circles both click wise and counter clock wise

3. Side to Side- this is a technique of vigorous shaking of the foot, gently to help circulation and relaxes the ankle and calf muscles.

4. Loosen Ankle- Hook both palms above the backside of the ankle so palm over the bones. Move hands rapidly back and forth in opposite directions. The foot will shake from side to side

5. Rotate all toes- This relaxation technique increases flexibility in toes and releases tension in the neck and shoulders.

6. Spinal twist- Grasp foot from the inside of the foot with both hands, finger on top. Uses both hands on a rocking motion, with the right hand twist up and down heal to toe.

7. Solar plexus breathing- with the hands on top of the foot squeeze in until you see and indentation, that is the solar plexus. Using both thumbs at the same time, finger o the back of the foot for leverage. Pushing in as the client breathes. Then release as the client exhales.

Crystals and Gemstones

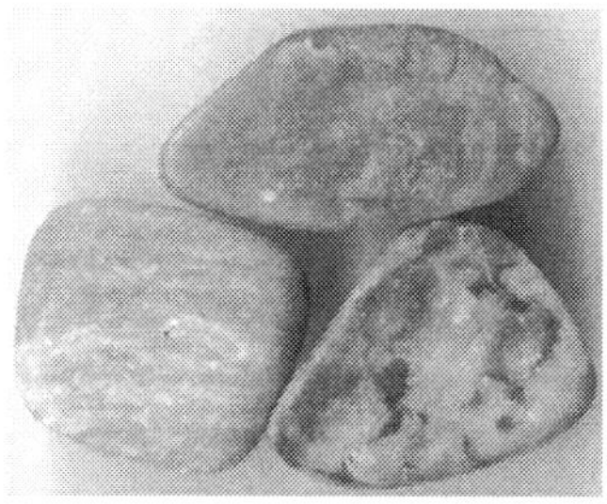

Preparing a Stone for Use

After you have chosen a stone to be used for healing, you need to cleanse it. Cleansing not only cleans the stone on the surface, but removes energetic residue that can linger from the store it came from, previous owners, people who may have touched it, or environmental vibrations it has absorbed along the way. You can do this in a number of simple ways. Choose whichever is most appealing to you:

*soak overnight in salted or sea/ocean water
*sit out overnight in the moonlight
*bury in dirt, salt, or sand for at least 1 hour
*sit in the sun for at least 1 hour (colored stones may fade so be careful here)
*wave through an incense, sage, or herbal blend designed for crystal clearing
*any other method you have learned elsewhere

Crystal Cleansing by Breath

In addition to many good methods for cleansing your crystals/stones using the Breath is a good choice. Sit with your stones/stones in front of you on the floor or table. Again, you know me I love doing things outside in nature but let that be your choice. Don't place them touching each other but rather given a little space to breathe. I usually place them in a circle. Bring now to your third eye, a golden/white flame. When you can see or "feel" it there take in a deep breath bringing the flame down from the third eye and pulling it into your mouth, hold the breath until you feel it's completed and then blow out over the stones. If there are several stones, I would suggest doing this a couple times. After you have completing the Breath, affirm mentally that all negative energies are cleared and give thanks to God/Spirit (or whomever you call to in prayer).

Programming a Stone

Once you have cleared the stone you will need to program it. What this does is focus the stone's energy for a specific purpose. As you will learn later on in the course, stones often have multiple properties it can be used for, so programming tells the stone what specific purpose you need it to do for you at this time. This isn't a permanent action, as you can cleanse and reprogram a stone an unlimited amount of times.

This is a very simple process. Hold the gem in your hand to sense its energy. Then take the stone and visualize the healing property you would like for it to have. As an example, let's say you want an amethyst to overcome depression. Picture in your mind's eye the amethyst absorbing anti-depressant energies. See the stone having the ability to stabilize emotions. Know that this will happen when you use the stone. When you feel that the programming is done, place in a box or other container or pouch. It is ready to be used.

One of the primary uses of stones is to balance the chakras. Chakra is an ancient Sanskrit word meaning wheel. The chakra system is a series of 7 energy centers that run from the base of the spine to the top of the head. This is illustrated on the next page. They are spinning vortexes of energy and need to be vibrating at the same speed for optimum health.

Connected to each chakra is a series of bodily organs and functions it is responsible for. We briefly cover this information here for your basic understanding for gemwork, but if you would like to learn more, we do offer a separate class in chakra therapy which includes more in depth material and other methods in addition to stones to do an entire chakra balancing session using multiple techniques.

To balance a chakra with gems, all you need to do is simply place them in the appropriate areas and allow them to sit for about 15 minutes or until they fall off of the client, whichever comes first.

We have provided a stone for each of the seven chakras in your kit. After placing the stone on the chakra(s), it's perfectly fine to use other stones on other regions of the body, set up a grid, or use other holistic therapies on the client.

The Chakra System

1. ROOT CHAKRA is at the base of the spine at the tailbone. You can visualize it in the area between the rectum and genitalia. I have found it is best to place the stone just between the legs of the client on the floor or table rather than invade the privacy of the person. Some practitioners prefer to place the stone on the very low abdomen. The root chakra is what grounds us, what ties us to the earth, and as such is the basis of our material issues. If the area is blocked or underactive the following may manifest in the client: fear, anxiety, obesity and weight issues including anorexia and eating disorders, insecurities, financial difficulties, and even knee, hip, leg, and lower back trouble. In men this is their sexual center, so any sexual dysfunction is attributed here. Stones to use here will be red in color, such as garnet, red **jasper**, red calcite, red tiger's eye, or any other deep red stone that appeals to you.

2. SACRAL CHAKRA is the second chakra and is located in the lower abdomen below the belly button. This is the region of female sexual energy, as well as sexual needs in both men and women. It is the area of creativity, intuition, self-worth, friendliness, and emotions. It is highly influenced buy how we were encouraged to express ourselves in early childhood. If blocked it may influence anger, manipulative behavior, sexual obsession or lack of desire, and reduced energy. Physical symptoms include kidney weakness, stiff lower back, constipation, ovulation or other menstrual irregularities, and muscle spasms. Overactive sacral symptoms- irritable bowel, diarrhea, frequent menstrual cycles, overactive bladder. Stones to use: any orange stone, such as **carnelian**, orange calcite, or sunstone.

3. SOLAR PLEXUS is the region in the middle of the stomach. This is best known for "gut instinct" so you are probably aware of your solar plexus. This is the center of your personal power, the ego, passions, and inner strength. It is also the center of astral travel, receptivity of spirit guides, and psychic development. If out of balance you may manifest lack of confidence, confusion, worried too much about what others think, feel out of control of your life, depression. Physical ailments include digestive disturbances, liver and detoxification problems, diabetes, nervous exhaustion, and food allergies. In balance it promotes cheerfulness, self-respect, freedom of expression, and a strong sense of personal power. This chakra controls the stomach, liver, gall bladder, pancreas, and small intestines, so depending on active these organs are tells you if the chakra is in balance, underactive, or

overactive. Stones to use would be any that are yellow, such as **citrine**, yellow jasper, **tiger's eye**, and pyrite.

4. HEART CHAKRA is located behind the breastbone. This is the center of love and emotions. It is here where one feels divine, unconditional love from the Creator/Universe. Here one learns to love self and others, connect compassionately and spiritually with others. This chakra connects body mind and spirit. Since almost everyone has a broken, hardened, or injured heart, this area needs special attention. When this chakra is out of balance, you may feel sorry for yourself, become paranoid, afraid to let go, feel unloved, and incapable of sending love to others. Physical ailments include heart attack/trouble, high blood pressure, insomnia, and difficulty breathing. The areas ruled by this chakra include the heart, lungs, circulation, shoulders, and upper back. Overactive heart chakras may cause heart palpitations, hyperactivity, too quick to fall in love or too clutching in a relationship. The colors are green or pink. Stones recommended include **rose quartz**, any pink stone, **green quartz**, aventurine, jade, or any green stone.

5. THROAT CHAKRA is located in the V in the collarbone and is the center of communication. Here one develops his or her own voice, their creative expression, music/sound, speech and writing. The possibility of change is controlled here. When out of balance, you will want to hold back, feel timid, be quiet, unable to express thoughts. Physical ailments include ear infections, sore throat, hyperthyroid, skin irritations/rashes, back pain, and general inflammation. In balance, you feel centered, well spoken, artistically inspired, and a clear communicator. Overactive signs are overly talkative, needing to speak without listening to others, scattered thoughts and speech. The body regions controlled by this chakra are the throat, neck, teeth, ears, and thyroid gland. Stones to use: any light to medium blue stone including **blue lace agate**, blue tiger's eye, aquamarine, turquoise.

6. THE THIRD EYE chakra is located in the center of your forehead. This is the center of psychic ability, higher intuition, and the energies of spirit and light. This area assists in the purification of negativity, elimination of selfish desires, and helps us to receive guidance. When in balance you are able to communicate with your higher self. When out of balance you my feel afraid of success, egoistic, or non-assertive. You will also feel alone and unable to communicate with your self. Physical illnesses include headaches, blurred vision, eyestrain, and even blindness. Overactive symptoms include oversensitivity to others, being overwhelmed psychically, or visions that you cannot understand. In balance you will find increased astral travel, telepathy,

interest in understanding past lives, and non-attachment to material things. It controls the eyes, face, brain, lymphatic system, and endocrine system. The stone color would be deep blue or purple, such as **sodalite**, lapis lazuli, **amethyst**, ametrine.

7. THE CROWN CHAKRA is located just above the top of the skull. This is the center of all spirituality and divine understanding. Here we gain wisdom and the gift of cosmic consciousness. The silver cord of the astral body connects to the crown. This is where the soul enters the body, and where it leaves at death. When unbalanced it causes frustration, no spark of joy, destructive tendencies, feeling alone in the universe. Physical illnesses include migraines and depression. When balanced you may be able to open up to Divine communication through channeling, dreams, etc. The color of the stone would be clear or milky white and can include **clear quartz** crystal, **moonstone**, or selenite.

Preparing for a Session

Before you begin, it is highly recommended that you do some form of a grounding meditation. Grounding helps the practitioner focus his or her energies and leave behind the worries of the day to day in order to shift our consciousness to the higher needs of the client. This can be done with any form of visualization that you may be familiar with. Even Yoga or tai Chi can be an excellent grounding meditation. If you don't already have a method of grounding, try the one below:

Find a quiet place and prepare it for a relaxing mood. You may sit or stand for this exercise. Candles, incense, and music can be added for mood enhancement. Close your eyes and pretend that you are a tree with very deep roots into the ground. Feel that your feet are the roots, and move upwards. Your arms and head are the foliage. Imagine that you are surrounded with a comforting white light. Feel connected to the earth, strong and solid. When you feel relaxed and that this has happened, take your time and open your eyes.

Laying on of Stones

The technique of using stones on a recipient's body for healing is called the laying on of stones. This powerful method cleansing the body, clears and balances the chakras, even stabilizes emotions and worries. Use only clean, cleared, programmed stones. The process can contain all quartz or any combination of stones for desired results. You can use stones you already own that were not provided in this course.

You can combine Reiki or any other holistic therapy with gem therapy. Place the stones starting from the head and work downward. Use gemstones that correspond with the chakras, then other stones to correct other illness in the body.
The energy of the stones need to flow in the same direction. Make sure all of the points face the same direction. If you wish to enlighten and uplift the recipient, make sure that the energy flows from down to up, earth to sky. If you wish to ground the recipient, then face the points down from sky to earth.

Therapeutic Gemstone Properties

Agate: Protection, good luck, balance body/mind/spirit, perceptiveness, strength, inspiration, awaken talents. Healing lore: Insomnia, teeth, gums, stomach problems, stamina, insomnia.

Amazonite: Integrity, success, joy, honor, creativity, self-esteem, calming, stress, self-destructive behaviors, psychic abilities. Healing lore: preventive, general health, heart problems, muscles, nervous system, tooth decay, osteoporosis.

Amber: Soothing, calming, cleansing, remove toxins, wisdom, purifying, intellect. Healing lore: Purify body, remove toxins, addictions, alcoholism, stress and anxiety related problems, poison, bone problems, heart problems, circulation, ears, hearing problems, endocrine system, fibromyalgia, intestinal/digestive disorders, kidney, bladder, lungs, general healing.

Amethyst: "Sobriety Stone", Peace, Calm, Inner Strength, Spirituality, Psychic Abilities, Dreamwork, Legal Problems, Money Issues; Healing lore - addictions, alcoholism, headaches, insomnia, arthritis, pain relief, circulatory system issues, endocrine system problems, chronic fatigue, fibromyalgia, immune system deficiencies, and general healing.

Ametrine: Intellectual stimulation, attunement, optimism, remove negative energy, releasing, dispelling tension, connecting, psychic abilities, remove prejudice, inner peace. Healing lore: Boost immune system, chronic fatigue syndrome, blood cleanser, repair DNA/RNA, depression.

Apatite: Intellect, achieving results, healing, insight, humanitarianism, meditation, balance, creativity. Healing lore: Bones, form new cells, calcium absorption, teeth, cartilage, suppress appetite, raises metabolism.

Aquamarine: Courage, luck, purification, peace, intuition, inner strength, self-expression, balance, relieve fear, calms communication, angel communication, preparedness, protection during travel on water. Healing lore: throat, speech, chronic fatigue, eyes, eyesight, fluid retention, headaches, intestinal /digestive.

Aventurine: Healing, money, mental agility, see potentials, happiness, peace, opening heart, creativity, imagination, motivation, leadership, friendship, gambling luck, good fortune, career success, protection. Healing lore: Strong healing, vision (physical), blood, headaches, sleep disorders, circulatory system.

Azurite: "Stone of Heaven", intuition, dreams, healing, insight, stilling the mind, concentration, self transformation, meditation, control energy. Healing lore: Prevent cancer, liver, arthritis, joints, depression, sinuses, skin.

Black Tourmaline: Ground excess energy, purifying, transform negative energy, protection, protection from black magick and the evil eye, deflect radiation from electronics, dispel fear. Healing lore: Obsessions, neuroses, emotional stability, immune system, heart disease, arthritis, brain tumors, gout.
Bloodstone: Courage, survival, adaptability, release blockages, renewal, strength, victory, intuitive decision making, abundance. Healing lore: Intense healing, emotional trauma, anemia, blood diseases, blood pressure, cardiovascular system, endocrine system, kidney, bladder, physical trauma, post-surgical recovery.

Blue Lace Agate: Tranquility, grace, higher spiritual planes, calming, gentleness, ease communication, public speaking, perform miracles, protection. Healing lore: Arthritis, headaches, digestive issues, growth, and bones.

Calcite: Amplify energy, lessen fear, reduce stress, purification, peace, calming, memory, awareness, appreciation of nature. Healing lore: Health, general healing, physical energy, back pain, physical strength, teeth, bones.

Carnelian: Creativity, manifestation, good luck, precision, analytical capabilities, verbal skill, protection, protection from anger, jealousy and fear, peace, spirituality, reduce sorrow. Healing lore: Open sores, rejuvenates tissues and cells, rheumatism, kidney stones, other kidney problems, gall stones, colds, pollen allergies, neuralgia.

Celestite: Angelic connection, verbal skill, healing, compassion, calming, growth, intuition, hope, emotional protection, decrease negativity. Healing lore: Eyes, mental disorders, eliminate toxins, digestion, cellular disorder.

Chrysocolla: Easing heartache, harmony, stamina, wisdom, peace, love, communication, vitality, inner strength, purify a place, remove negativity, reduce fear anxiety and guilt. Healing lore: Asthma, TB, pneumonia, muscle cramps, arthritis, childbirth, pregnancy.

Chrysoprase: Good fortune, prosperity, balance male-female energy, love, grace, compassion, clemency, personal growth, mend broken heart. Healing lore: Eyesight, eyes, immune system, fertility, gout, mental illness, fevers, excess body heat, sexually transmitted disease.

Citrine: Success, intuition, comfort, creativity, physical energy, wealth, mental awakening, protection, good fortune / luck, decrease nightmares, remove toxins. Healing lore: Depression, mood swings, trauma, grief, digestion, stomach, eliminating nightmares and other sleep disturbances, thyroid, general health, heart, kidney, liver, muscles, strength, endocrine system, circulatory system, tissue regeneration, urinary system, immune system, fibromyalgia, addictions, OCD.

Clear Quartz (Crystal Quartz, Rock Crystal): Power stone, Intensify energy, spiritual development, healing, raising consciousness, counter black magic. Healing lore: Master Healer, diagnostics, pain, arthirtis, bone injuries, depression, fibromyalgia, intestines, mental and physical energy, stamina, physical strength.

Coral: Diplomacy, wonders of nature, creativity, optimism, understanding of purpose, quieting emotions, visualization. Healing lore: General healing, blood, circulatory system, kidney, bladder, epilepsy, bone, bone marrow, eyes, respiratory system.

Dumortierite: Self-reliance, mental clarity, stamina, patience, recognition of potential, understanding, communication of ideas, spiritual development. Healing lore: Throat, thyroid, parathyroid, detoxification, overstimulation, blood, spleen, hyperactivity, endocrine system.

Emerald: Love, domestic bliss, sensitivity, loyalty, memory, mental capacity, harmony, focus, eliminating negativity, romance, memory, faith, truthfulness. Healing lore: Remove mental causes of disease and unwellness, disease, general healing.

Fluorite: Stability, peace and calm, impartial reasoning, responsibility, concentration, spiritual wholeness, psychic development, meditation, mental blocks, aura cleansing, protection from psychic attack, self-love. Healing lore: Health, skeletal system, muscular system.

Fossils: Accomplishments, improvement of one's environment, business, communication, innovation, get rid of old habits, quality, telepathic. Healing lore: Paranoia, schizophrenia, long life, abuse recovery.

Garnet: Remove negativity, romantic love, passion, sensuality, intimacy, career success, self-confidence, protection from evil, awareness, commitment, regeneration, order, insight. Healing lore: Health, cellular regeneration, blood, heart, lungs.

Hematite: Mental attunement, memory, calming, balance, grounding, centering, focusing energy and emotions, peace, inner happiness, transforming negativity. Healing lore: keep the body cool, blood disorders, nervous problems, insomnia, align the spine, mend broken bones, anemia.

Howlite: Awareness, calm, emotional expression, observation, patience, eliminating negativity, selfishness, creativity. Healing lore: Bones, teeth, calcium levels, leg cramps.

Infinite: Infinite is a name for a variety of green serpentine found in South Africa. Its energies are believed to be superior to those of other serpentines and it has come to be known as the "Healer's Stone". It repatterns the auric field and is a well used stone for Reiki and other energy therapies. It can activate the kundalini and has been reported to help heal AIDS, cancer, and other serious/terminal diseases. The unique energy of Infinite works on all levels of the self. It stimulates physical, emotional and spiritual healing and makes an excellent tool for the healing of loss, separation and betrayal. It is a beneficial grief stone. This stone also aids in the connection to the Angelic realms.

Iolite (aka Water Sapphire): Intuition, spiritual growth, balance, releasing discord, awakening to inner knowledge, Shaman stone, visions. Healing lore: Strong healing, addictions, sobriety, detoxification, sore throat, varicose veins, blisters.

Jade: Fidelity, dreams, realization of potential, peace, accord, resourcefulness, accomplishment, emotional balance, protection. Healing lore: Heart, illness, kidneys.

Jaspers: Protection, nurturing, joy, awareness, relaxation, tranquility, wholeness, astral travel, Yin/Yang. Healing lore: Liver, gallbladder, stomach.

Jet: Grief, mourning, protection from evil negativity and psychic attacks, financial safety, depression, sympathy. Healing lore: epilepsy, migraines, stomach pain, colds, glandular problems, lymphatic problems.

Labradorite: Alignment, attract success, dreams, reduce stress and anxiety, spiritual connection.

Lapis: Manifestation, wisdom, truthfulness, openness, communication, inner power, intuition, spiritual evolution, virility, self-confidence, objectivity, dreams, purity, serenity, guardian spirits, love & fidelity within marriage, protection. Healing lore: Sinus ailments, insomnia, depression, recurring fevers, vision, hearing, throat, lungs, immune system.

Lepidolite: Hope, stress reduction, birth, peace, acceptance, spirituality, physical strength, luck, protection, emotional balance. Healing lore: Bipolar disorder, stress, anxiety, depression, manic depression, despondency, PTSD, anger, traumas, panic attacks, addictions, glands, immune system, skin, nails, hair, DNA, enzyme balance, alcoholism recovery, pregnancy, childbirth, general healing.

Malachite: Transformation, insight, spiritual evolution, protection during pregnancy and childbirth, clarifying emotions, fidelity, loyalty, practicality. Healing lore: Radiation sickness, asthma, arthritis, tumors.

Onyx: Self-control, decision making, conquer challenges, intuition, recognition of personal strengths, grounding, protection. Healing lore: Stamina, childbirth, wound healing.

Opal: Creativity, inspiration, hope, spontaneity, relationships, memory, happy dreams, changes. Healing, Eyesight, Parkinson's disease, depression.

Peridot: Warmth, friendliness, understanding, openness in love and relationships, regulation of cycles, ESP, find what is lost, protective shield. Healing lore: High healing energy, slow aging, ulcers, digestion problems.

Pietersite: Relaxation, relieve worries, courage, improve memory, tenacity, work with angels, astral travel, release deep emotions calmly. Healing lore: Body fluid balance, nutrition, gastrointestinal functions, endocrine glands, female hormones, PMS, menopause.

Pyrite (Fool's Gold, Healer's Gold): Defense, prevention, protection from negativity, leadership, psychic abilities, memory, shields from physical danger. Healing lore: Physical wholeness, lungs, inflammations, stamina, digestion, circulation.

Rhodocrosite: Love, emotional balance, "Stone of Love and Balance", cleansing, renewal, relaxation, expansion of consciousness. Healing lore: Digestion, kidneys, thyroid, pulse rate, digestion.

Rhodonite: Grace, elegance, peace, generosity, attention to details, calming, unconditional love, service to mankind. Healing lore: Emphysema, joint inflammation, light sensitivity, strep throat, heart disorders.

Rhyolite: Change, variety, progress, creativity, transcending barriers, Yin/Yang. Healing lore: Liver cleansing, throat, general healing.

Rose Quartz: Love of all kinds including self-love, protection during pregnancy and childbirth, peace, happiness, gentleness. Healing lore: Emotional wounds, heart, the circulatory system, fertility, headaches, kidney disease, migraines, sexual dysfunction, sinus problems, throat problems, depression, addictions, ear aches, slows signs of aging in general, reduces wrinkles, spleen problems, fibromyalgia, and reaching one's ideal weight / weight loss.

Ruby: Integrity, generosity, nurturing, spiritual wisdom, attainment of values, economic stability and prosperity, protection from distress, home and contents protection. Healing lore: Emotional problems, fever, constrictions in circulatory system, heart, blood flow, muscular system, throat, parathyroid glands, brain.

Sapphire: Joy, peace, beauty, creative expression, meditation, intuition, prosperity, fulfillment of dreams, mental clarity. Healing lore: Relieve depression, lower fevers, reduce inflammation, burns, hearing problems.

Serpentine ("New Jade"): Attract love and money, emotional cleansing, psychic powers, kundalini rising, protection from snakebite, poison and venom, meditation, restore self-confidence. Healing: Parasitic infections, snakebite, venom and other poisons, cellular regeneration, balance female hormones, milk production in nursing mothers.

Silver Topaz: Soul mirror, intuition, psychic, improve speech, eloquence, enhance and store energies of gemstones, draw out negative energies, moon energies, feminine/yin energy. Healing lore: Hepatitis, eliminate toxins, headache, rheumatic pain, nausea, gastritis, obesity, diabetes, increase assimilation of vitamins A and E.

Smoky Quartz: Dissolving emotional blockage, clearing the mind, cooperation, grounding and centering, personal pride, joy in living, attentiveness to the moment, protection, good luck. Healing lore: Kidneys, abdomen, pancreas, reproductive organs, menstrual cramps, fertility issues, water retention.

Sodalite: Wisdom, logic, calmness, healing, stress reduction, companionship, self-esteem, work in groups, heal communication breeches, truth, intelligence, knowledge, learning. Healing lore: Glands, digestive system, insomnia, calcium deficiency, head colds.

Sunstone: Alleviating fears & phobias, energizing, cleansing, "Leadership Stone", decrease stress and depression, personal power, life force energy, animal guides, spirit guides. Healing lore: general health, physical energy, sexual dysfunction, increase sexual energy.

Tanzanite: "Workaholic's Stone", Communication, intuition, protection, symmetry, decision-making, spirituality, slow down and take it easy, relieve stress, composure, harmony, poise. Healing lore: Stress related illness, high blood pressure.

Tiger Eye: Self- discipline, practicality, protection, grounding peacefulness, clarity, intelligence, intuition & psychic powers, new experiences, financial stability, calmness, releasing inhibitions, integrity, willpower, prosperity, personal power, kundalini. Healing lore: Heal wounds, bruises, colon, digestion, stomach problems, eyes, night vision, reduce pain, alcoholism, reproductive system.

Turquoise: Spiritual attunement, cleansing, communication, healing, protection, valor, soothing, peace of mind, guidance through the unknown, romantic spontaneity. Healing lore: "Master Healing Stone", prevents illness, bipolar disorder, panic disorder, all health issues in general.

Unakite: Balance, re-birth, foresight, emotional balance, release blockages. Healing lore: Reproductive system, healthy pregnancy, development of unborn child.

How to Conduct a Session

Before you begin to work on your client, make sure to prepare the room. You may wish to use a smudge or incense designed for purification such as sage, frankincense, sandalwood, or cedar. Make sure that the room is empowered with healing energy. This space should be quiet, comfortable and the right temperature. Invoke and invite any spirit guides or ascended masters, if desired. Call upon your Highest Self to help you with the healing.

The client need not remove any clothing other than shoes. Jewelry can stay on if desired. Start with a clear quartz above the head and a hematite or other dark grounding stone at the feet to place the polarities. Next, scan their auric field to see if you feel temperature differences. You can use a stone, a wand, or your hand for the scanning.

You can do a session face to face with a client, or via distance with the help of their photo or using meditation or visualization.

Office Sessions

The crystals and stones can be placed

1. ***Upon the subject in a grid or pattern.***
   Be extra careful when placing crystals or stones in particularly sensitive areas such as eyelids.
   You can use a pre-planned grid or pattern, or place the stones on the chakras, or use your intuition to access healing information from the Divine and use a pattern of your own devising.

2. ***Below the subject.***
   Again, you can use pre-planned grids or patterns or use your intuition.
   Be careful of accidentally causing stone bruises, and pad the stones if necessary when placing them under the client.

3. ***Around him or her.***
   Near or touching the body in a pattern around the client can work well for healing.
   You can effectively make the client part of the pattern in this way.

Distance Sessions

You can use a substitute to stand in for the actual client who is at a distance from you. A photograph of the client is a great substitute, however, if no photo is available, writing down their name and using that is good also.

Next, go chakra to chakra, starting with the feet and working up. Place the appropriate chakra stone on each center. (Place the stones near you before the session). As you place the stone, visualize the color of that chakra. Flick your fingers over the chakra to release any built up or negative energy.

Have other stones available- you never know which stones may call out to you until you begin. Have as many crystals and gemstones in your collection as you can. Your assortment will grow in time. If you place a stone and it quickly rolls off, let it stay off. DO NOT HOLD A STONE IN AN AREA THAT IS REJECTING IT. If the body does not need a stone it will fall off. You may also see this happen in the chakras. THERE ARE NO SET RULES IN LAYING THE STONES. If the recipient is uncomfortable with any stone or having a stone in any area, remove it.

Finish with brushing the aura, either with a feather or your own hands. Sweep about 3 to 6 "above the body from head to toe in a slow, deliberate, gentle motion.

Another option for you is to simply place the stones, then wait for the gems to do their work. The stones will roll off one by one as the chakras and subtle bodies absorb their energies. This method can take a lot longer and patience is required. It relies on the healer's intuition to know when to remove the stones. It may work well when dealing with distant healings or when an intense session is required.

Remove the stones one by one. Do not use these stones again until they have been cleared. I place them in rock salt in a large plastic divided container used to sort office supplies. You can use any method that works for you.

The laying of stones can be a very intense experience…there are often major energy shifts. Allow the client time to rest before leaving the healing session. It is possible for past life, forgotten trauma, or other deep-rooted issues to surface. A healer must remain neutral and detached from the outcome. Allow them to experience their pain, joy, or peace fully. Listen to what they share with you. Be compassionate and understanding. Keep what they tell you in confidence.

Other Uses for Gemstones

Quartz and other stones can be added to fish tanks, inside planters, in the car, on top of the computer, or any place where you want to add their type of energy. I keep a malachite in the cash register at all times, an amethyst and quartz in each corner of the healing room, and I never go out without carrying a small pouch of chakra stones with me. Rose quartz is wonderful for helping depression, malachite for toothaches, amethyst for meditation, etc.

Experiment with each stone to see how it feels to you. Be very selective and take your time when buying a new gem.

Grids and Layouts

A Grid is a way to arrange stones in a specific pattern and is seen as an advanced gemstone layout. A layout is a random laying out of stones for a situation (for instance gathering malachite, green tourmaline, and jade for money and placing them on your bed stand is a layout. Arranging a set array of stones on the flower of life pattern in this course would be a grid, as it is believed how you place the stones is what gives a grid its power.)

Grids are consciously activated by connecting a line of Light between the stones so that they vibrate their energy in the environment in which they are set up. To activate a Grid, use your finger, a wand if you have one, or one of those larger gemstone laser wands that you might have been seeing in stores and wondering what they were used for, they are used for grids (and other uses as well I am sure!). However I have always found that your own finger or intuition in activating a grid is the best tool.

Grids can be placed in an environment or used in healing, when they are used environment they are just placed somewhere safe and activated. When they are used in healing they may be placed beneath the person or on them depending which grids are used. I like to use smaller stones when placing them on someone, they stay neater.

Smudging your area before and after would be a good idea because there will be a lot of 'release' in the room you don't want hanging around. To smudge light some sage start in one corner of the room and go from wall to wall back to the starting spot, see the room full of Light and clear as the smoke swirls.
I chose these stones for their properties and they are also some of the stones I've used for my Healing Therapy Course. Use 7 stones of each and arrange in a 'Star of David' pattern or a upward and then downward pointing triangle.

Draw a line from the first stone to the center then back to the next stone and back to the center, making a wheel like pattern. The geometric pattern creates a radiating of energy, this is done through a spiral vortex in both an upward, downward and outward direction at the location of the Grid itself. If you are sensitive to energy you will be able to feel right away that there is a shift of frequency in the room where you set up a grid.

Clearing your space, often called “smudging” or space clearing in Feng Shui, can be very helpful when setting up a grid. You can however open the windows, use energy/Reiki, prayer, meditation, or any other practice that suits your beliefs and skill level to prepare the room prior to setting up the grid.

On the following page are specific directions to set up a grid. You can follow them or use your inner guidance to create one that suits your needs.

How to Create a Grid

1. Ask your guides to assist you in locating the appropriate crystals. Some of these may be amethyst and rose quartz crystals too.

2. Wash them in sea salt, the purest you can find and allow them to dry, preferably in the sun.

3. Place them one at a time in your hands and telepathically send them your intentions. Remember your intentions are their instructions telling them what kind of energy wave to emit into the grid.

4. Ask them where they would like to be placed and then allow them to guide you to that destination. You will know by feeling. They communicate telepathically and emotionally. You will know that you found the right place for them because it will *feel* really good to you.

How to Maintain a Grid

- Pick them up and talk to them often. Remember they are little people in crystal bodies and they need love and attention just like we do.

- Grids can be set up for short term use such as for the length of a healing session, or long term for chronic conditions, attracting prosperity, protection, or as a study aide to give a few examples

- Send Reiki, positive thoughts, and/or prayers to the grid regularly to enhance its energies.

Birthstones by Color and Month

January: dark red Garnet

February: purple Amethyst

March: pale blue Aquamarine

April: clear Diamond

May: green Emerald

June: cream Pearl, Moonstone

July: red Ruby

August: light green Peridot

September: blue Sapphire

October: multi-tonal Opal, Tourmaline

November: yellow Citrine, yellow Topaz

December: Turquoise, Blue Topaz, Blue Zircon, Tanzanite

Gemstones for Common Conditions

1. Acidity	Aventurine+ Citrine
2. Accidents	Red Jasper+ Obsidian
3. Arthritis,	Red Jasper + Carnelian + Citrine
4. Asthma	Blue Lace Age + Sodalite
5. Bronchitis, Common Cold, &Throat	Red Jasper
6. Cancer	Blue Lace Agate + Red Jasper
7. Digestive Disorder	Carnelian +Citrine
8. Ear troubles	Red Jasper + Blue Lace Agate
9. Eczema & skin conditions, acne	Amethyst + Moonstone
10.Epilepsy, seizures, spasms	Aventurine + Moon Stone
11 Goiter and glandular balance	Obsidian + Blue Lace Agate
12.General illness, not yet determined	Red Coral+ Moonstone
13.Heart Disease	Aventurine
14. High Blood Pressure	Aventurine+ Sodalite
15. Impatience/ unable to relax	Amethyst + Sodalite
16. Insomnia & sleep disorders	Amethyst + Moonstone + Sodalite
17. Irritable Bowel/ intestinal issues	Quartz + Bloodstone
18. Leukemia/Blood diseases	Hematite + Bloodstone + Quartz
19. Menstrual Disorders/female issues	Moonstone + Carnelian
20. Mental Illness/Stress	Amethyst + Rose Quartz
21. Men's Health Issues	Red Jasper + Carnelian+ Quartz
22. Migraines/Headaches	Amethyst + Quartz
23. Overcome Addictions	Amethyst + Rose Quartz + Sodalite
24. Pain Relief	Quartz, Obsidian, Amethyst
25. Protection	Obsidian + Quartz
26. Psychic Enhancement	Amethyst, Moonstone, Sodalite
27. Urinary/Bladder Conditions	Carnelian + Hematite
28. Wealth/Prosperity	Aventurine + Citrine
29. Weight Loss	Blue Lace Agate + Moonstone+ Amethyst

What are Gem Elixirs/Essences

Gem essences are specially prepared vibrational remedies, which are used to alleviate mild emotional conditions. Gem essences work on a similar basis as homeopathic and flower essence remedies, using the subtle vibrations of gems and stones to effect a positive transition in one's emotional or spiritual life. Gem essences are sometimes called elixirs to not confuse an essence with an aroma. They are often called elixirs, and the terms essences and elixirs are used interchangeably.

The Vibration of Gem Elixirs

"Gem Elixir" is the name given to a fluid that has been infused with the energies of a crystal, either through the power of sunlight or moonlight. Water has the ability to hold energy patterns intact for long periods of time, therefore making this an ideal medium for capturing the powers of a stone. Sunlight is traditionally used for elixirs that are designed for aiding the physical body, whereas moonlight is used for those that are directed towards spiritual and magickal needs. These elixirs can then be used for healing, magick, or just whenever you need to take in the energies of a particular crystal or gem.

Place your crystal or gem in the bowl/glass, and cover with the pure water. Simply place this in an area that will be exposed to the direct sun/moon for your selected period of time.. If you are able to sit it on the roof of your house, this is a good spot, as it catches the rays from all angles, and is less likely to have any shadows pass over it during the infusion process.

Leave the infusion untouched for at least the 3 hours, then pour the liquid into the clean dark glass bottle. Half fill the bottle with your infusion, and then top up the rest of the bottle with brandy, or another spirit. The alcohol content, when taken in the correct dosage is negligible, so you need not worry about this. If, however you are concerned, you can add your dose to very hot water, then wait for it to cool before drinking. This way, the alcohol evaporates with the heat, and you are left with absolutely no alcohol content. Seal the bottle, and then shake vigorously for 30 seconds.

Elixirs can be administered directly under the tongue, undiluted, as with flower essences. The rich blood supply to the mouth area, and the thin skin under the tongue allows for rapid absorption of the elixir. You can also apply some to an afflicted area of the body that you are wishing to treat, or use in a bath.

Herbalism

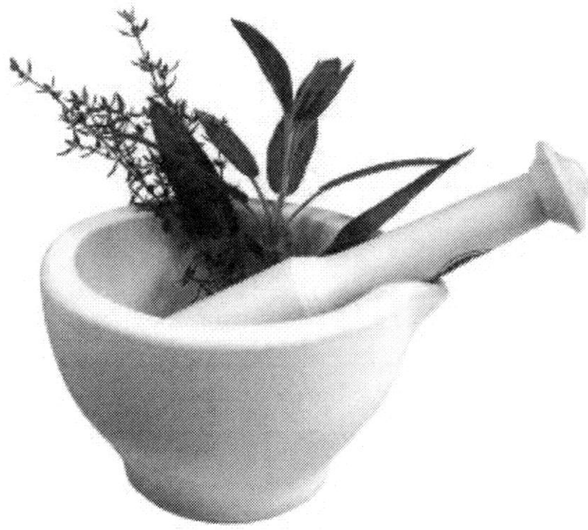

Herbal Medicine, sometimes referred to as Herbalism or Botanical Medicine, is the use of herbs for their therapeutic or medicinal value. An herb is a plant or plant part valued for its medicinal, aromatic or savory qualities. Herb plants produce and contain a variety of chemical substances that act upon the body.

Herbal medicine is the oldest form of healthcare known to mankind. Herbs had been used by all cultures throughout history. It was an integral part of the development of modern civilization. Primitive man observed and appreciated the great diversity of plants available to him. The plants provided food, clothing, shelter, and medicine. Much of the medicinal use of plants seems to have been developed through observations of wild animals, and by trial and error. As time went on, each tribe added the medicinal power of herbs in their area to its knowledgebase. They methodically collected information on herbs and developed well-defined herbal pharmacopoeias.

Indeed, well into the 20th century much of the pharmacopoeia of scientific medicine was derived from the herbal lore of native peoples. Many drugs commonly used today are of herbal origin such as valium from valerian root as a common example. Indeed, about 25 percent of the prescription drugs dispensed in the United States contain at least one active ingredient derived from plant material. Some are made from plant extracts; others are synthesized to mimic a natural plant compound. This is why herbs and pharmaceuticals can and often do have interactions if taken together. This course can not possibly go into detail on interactions, as there are volumes of books written just to cover them all. I highly suggest if you plan to work with herbs on a regular basis, especially if you decide to work with others, that you purchase a book on herb, drug, and supplement interactions. They are readily available at almost all bookstores and are published by many reputable authors.

The World Health Organization (WHO) estimates that 4 billion people, 80 percent of the world population, presently use herbal medicine for some aspect of primary health care. Herbal medicine is a major component in all indigenous peoples' traditional medicine and a common element in Ayurvedic, homeopathic, naturopathic, traditional oriental, and Native American Indian medicine. WHO notes that of 119 plant-derived pharmaceutical medicines, about 74 percent are used in modern medicine in ways that correlated directly with their traditional uses as plant medicines by native cultures. Major pharmaceutical companies are currently conducting extensive research on plant materials gathered from the rain forests and other places for their potential medicinal value.

Substances derived from the plants remain the basis for a large proportion of the commercial medications used today for the treatment of heart disease, high blood pressure, pain, asthma, and other problems. For example, ephedra is a herb used in Traditional Chinese Medicine for more than two thousand years to treat asthma and other respiratory problems. Ephedrine, the active ingredient in ephedra, is used in the commercial pharmaceutical preparations for the relief of asthma symptoms and other respiratory problems. It helps the patient to breathe more easily. Due to its highly stimulating qualities, its been readily used in diet drugs, a misuse to say the least although it can be affective. However, this herb, like any other herb, can be abused, can cause allergies, and can create side effects. There were a number of cases of heart attacks and even death from dieters who fasted, took ephedra based products, and performed strenuous exercise, so this herb was deemed unsafe by the FDA and banned in most forms. While I do understand the rationale, it is now out of the hands of most trained herbalists, even the skilled Chinese medicine practitioners who know exactly how to dose a client with allergies, asthma, and other respiratory conditions. It's a shame that the lack of knowledge of herbalism has not only harmed innocent people, but can keep these natural remedies out of the hands of countless others whose lives could be drastically improved with its inclusion. Please approach herbs with respect, logic, and understanding, as they are medicines and can be overdosed like any other drug.

Herbal Medicine can be broadly classified into various basic systems: Traditional Chinese Herbalism, which is part of Traditional Oriental Medicine, Ayurvedic Herbalism, which is derived from Ayurveda, and Western Herbalism, which originally came from Greece and Rome to Europe and then spread to North and South America.

Chinese and Ayurvedic Herbalism have developed into highly sophisticated systems of diagnosis and treatment over the centuries. Western Herbalism is today primarily a system of folk medicine.

Interest in the United States had been growing in the recent years from the reported success stories from the use of herbs. For example, St. John's Wort is widely used in the treatment of mild depression without the need for Prozac. St. John's Wort does not have the side effects such as that of Prozac. There are some Ayurvedic herbs that are very useful for reducing cholesterol, diabetes etc. Similarly the popularity of Ginseng and Ginkgo biloba (ginkgo) is rising due to its beneficial effects.

Drug Regulation

Today in the United States, herbal products can be marketed only as food supplements. An herb manufacturer or distributor can make no specific health claims without FDA approval. Remember my ephedra reference from above? That is just the tip of the iceberg to say the least.

Two features of European drug regulation make that market more hospitable to natural remedies. First, it costs less and takes less time in Europe to approve medicines as safe and effective. This is especially true of substances that have a long use history and can be approved under the "doctrine of reasonable certainty." European guidelines for the assessment of herbal remedies follow up on WHO's Guidelines for the Assessment of Herbal Medicines, which state that a substance's historical use is a valid way to document safety and efficacy in the absence of scientific evidence to the contrary.

France, where traditional medicines can be sold with labeling based on traditional use, requires licensing by the French Licensing Committee and approval by the French Pharmacopoeia Committee. Germany considers whole herbal products one active ingredient; this makes it simpler to define and approve the product. The German Federal Health Office regulates products such as ginkgo and milk thistle extracts so that potency and manufacturing processes are standardized. England generally follows the rule of prior use; that is, years of use with apparent positive effects and no evidence of detrimental side effects constitute enough evidence---in lieu of other scientific data---that the product is safe.

In Japan, China, and India, patent herbal remedies composed of dried and powdered whole herbs or herb extracts, often in tablet form, are the rule. Traditional herbals are the backbone of China's medicine. Japan's traditional medicine, kampo, is similar to and historically derived from Chinese medicine but includes traditional medicines from Japanese folklore. Herbal medicines are the staple of medical treatment in many developing countries and are used for many types of ailments.

Standardized vs. Whole Herb

As the herbs are getting more and more popular, more and more manufacturers are supplying standardized herb extracts. A standardized extract means that the manufacturer has verified that the active ingredient believed to be present in the herb is present in the preparation and that the potency and the amount of the active ingredient is assured in the preparation. The problem is that, the action of the herb may be from a number of constituents and not from just one or two ingredients. Thus, the standardized preparation may omit some of the ingredients and we will lose out on the effect from the complex combination of the constituents.

Herb and Food Interactions

Many people have the mistaken notion that, being natural, all herbs and foods are safe. This is not so. Very often, herbs and foods may interact with medications you normally take that result in serious side reactions. It is always a good practice to tell your doctor or health practitioners what you are taking so that they can advise you of possible complications, if there is any. You should also keep an eye for unusual symptoms. Very often, this may foretell the symptoms of a drug interaction.

Experts suggest that natural does not mean it is completely safe. Everything you put in your mouth has the potential to interact with something else. The medication that is taken by mouth travels through the digestive system in much the same way as food and herbs taken orally do. So, when a drug is mixed with food or another herb, each can alter the way the body metabolizes the other. Some drugs interfere with the body's ability to absorb nutrients. Similarly, some herbs and foods can lessen or increase the impact of a drug.

As more and more people discover new herbs, there is more and more potential for the abuse of these herbs and the patients may end up in serious problems. For example, St. John's Wort has been shown to have great potential to control minor depression. The National Institutes of Health is conducting a clinical study to determine the effect of St. John's Wort scientifically. A customer at my store recently was of the mindset that if a little is good, a lot is better. Plus this particular herb can interact with MAO inhibitors as well as birth control pills, and she apparently was on both, and never told her doctor or pharmacist. It was me who caught the interaction before it was too late and advised her of other options. This is why I am a major advocate of educating customers prior to making the sale. While its not legal for non-doctors to treat or diagnose, I do feel there is a liability on behalf of a store or holistic healer if we do not gather information about the customer and help prevent misuse or interactions.

High-risk patients, such as the elderly, patients taking three or more medications for chronic conditions, patients suffering from diabetes, hypertension, depression, high cholesterol or congestive heart failure, should be especially on the lookout for such side reactions. Best bet, if you can, try to advise that they not begin an herbal regimen if they are taking any prescriptions unless they educate themselves. Ultimately the choice is theirs, but as a holistic practitioner or shopkeeper it is up to you to help empower them to make the best choice for their needs.

Glossary of Medicinal Properties Of Herbs

Abortifacient: Induces the premature abortion of the fetus. Example: pennyroyal, aloe, sandalwood.

Adaptogens: Herbs that help us adapt to stress by supporting the adrenal glands, the endocrine system, and the whole person. Examples are ginseng root, nettle leaf, sarsaparilla, licorice root, and ashwagandha.

Alterative:(Sanskrit: Parivartakas or Rakta Shodhana Karma) These herbs alter or change a long-standing condition by aiding the elimination of metabolic toxins. Gradually facilitates a beneficial change in the body. Also known as "blood cleansers' in the past, these herbs improve lymphatic circulation, boost immunity, and help clear chronic conditions of the skin. These herbs also heal sores, boils, tumors, cancers; reduces fevers; detoxifies the liver, kills parasites and worms; helps in the treatment of infectious, contagious diseases and epidemics, flu, acne herpes, and venereal disease. Examples are: ginseng, aloe, sandalwood, red clover, burdock, bayberry, black pepper, cinnamon, myrrh, and safflower.

Analgesic or Anodynes: (Sanskrit- Vedana shamana) These herbs reduce or eliminate pain (e.g., digestive, circulatory, respiratory, nervous system, nerve, muscle, tooth pain, nervous digestion, headaches). Some herbs are strong pain relievers, often working best against pains of specific causes. Examples: Camphor, chamomile, cinnamon, cloves, echinacea, lavender flower, feverfew herb, cabbage leaves, wintergreen leaf , passionflower herb and flower.

Anaphrodisiac: Herbs that decrease or allay sexual feelings or desires.

Anesthetics: For surgical anesthesia. Examples are: ashok, calamus, gudmar, and jatamanshi.

Antacid: Neutralizes the acid produced by the stomach. Helps the stomach lining recuperate to accommodate the healthy gastric acid needed for good digestion.

Examples are: marshmallow root and leaf, meadowsweet herb, hops flower, and sweet flag.

Antibiotic: Inhibits the growth of germs, bacteria, and harmful microbes. Examples: Turmeric and echinacea.

Antidiabetic: Examples of herbs: Amalaki, blackberry, fenugreek, gudmar, senna, and shilajit.

Antidiarrheal: An alterative. Examples are: Blackberry, comfrey, gentian, red raspberry, and yellow dock, black pepper, and ginger.

Antiemetic: (Sanskrit: Chherdinashana) Prevents or alleviates nausea and vomiting. Examples are: Cloves, coriander, ginger, and raspberry.

Antiseptic: (Sanskrit- Shodhaniya) prevents decay or putrefaction. A substance that inhibits the growth and development of microorganisms without necessarily destroying them. Also see bitter. Examples are: Aloe, Chitrak, gokshura, gudmar, sandalwood, and turmeric.

Antispasmodic: (Sanskrit- Vikashi) Relieves or prevents involuntary muscle spasm or cramps (also see nervines) by strengthening nerves and the nervous system. Examples: Camomile, ashwagandha, basil, calamus, guggul, licorice, myrrh, sage, gotu kola, jatamanshi, peppermint, sandalwood, and spearmint.

Aperient: (Sanskrit- Bhedaniya) A mild or gentle laxative. Also called aperitive. Example: Rhubarb.

Aphrodisiac: (Sanskrit- Vajikarana) Restores or increases sexual power and desire. Two types: Tonics: Develop tissue substance. Stimulants: increase the functioning of the reproductive organs. Examples: Angelica, ahwagandha, asparagus, fenugreek, fo-ti, ginseng, gokshura, hibiscus, kapikachu seeds, pippali, rose, saffron, and shatavari. The nutritive tonics such as aghwagandha, bala, fo-ti, ghee, licorice, marshmallow, sesame seeds, and Shatavari increase semen and breast milk.

Astringent: (Sanskrit- Sankeshanlya or Stambhana karma) Causes a local contraction of the skin, blood vessels, and other tissues, thereby arresting the discharge of blood, mucus, etc. Usually used locally as a topical application. Examples: Amalaki, arjuna, ashok, cinnamon, jasmine, sandalwood, and yarrow.

Bitter: a solution of bitter, often aromatic, plant products used as a mild tonic. These herbs reduce toxins, toxins in blood and weight, destroy infection, high fever, heat, fever in blood, internal fever, heated liver, much thirst, sweating, inflammation, and infection. Examples: aloe, barberry, chirayata, gentian, and golden seal.

Calmative: Herbs that are soothing, sedating-see also nervines.

Cardiac Stimulant: Herbs that promote circulation when there is a weak heart.

Carminative: (Sanskrit- Vata-anuloman or Dipaniya) Herb that helps to prevent gas from forming in the intestines, and also assists in expelling it. Also increases absorption of nutrients, dispels water, mucus, promotes normal peristalsis; relieves spasms and pain; improves weak digestion from anxiety, nervousness, or depression. Examples: Chamomile, chrysanthemum, coriander, fennel, lime, peppermint, and spearmint, ajwan, basil, calamus, cardamom, cinnamon, ginger, and turmeric.

Cathartic: (Sanskrit- Bhedana) Causes evacuation of the bowels. A cathartic may be either mild (laxative) or vigorous (purgative). Examples are: figs, prunes, olive oil (laxatives), senna, castor oil, and aloe vera.

Cholagogue: Herb that stimulates the flow of bile from the liver into the intestines. Examples: Arka, guduchi, licorice, safflower, senna, and sesame.

Decongestant: For relieving congestion-see expectorant.

Demulcent: (Sanskrit- Mridukara or Kasa-Svasahara) Soothes, protects, and relieves the irritation of inflamed mucous membranes and other surfaces. (i.e., protects stomach and urinary bladder lining). Examples: Barley, licorice; linseed, olive, and almond oils.

Diaphoretic: (Sanskrit- Svedana Karma or Svedaniya) Promotes perspiration, especially profuse perspiration. Promotes circulation; dispels fever and chills; eliminates surface toxins; relieves muscle tension, aching joints, and inflammatory skin conditions; relieves diarrhea, dysentery, kidneys, liver, urinary, and gall bladder disorders; dispels stones of kidney and both bladders. Also useful for genitourinary disease (herpes), edema; painful, difficult or burning urination or infections. See sudorific. Examples: basil, ajwan, cardamom, parsley, cinnamon, eucalyptus, ginger, juniper berries, asparagus, barley, burdock, chamomile, chrysanthemum, coriander, dandelion, fennel, marshmallow, spearmint.

Digestives: (Sanskrit- Dipana-Pachana Karma) Assists the stomach and intestines in normal digestion. Examples: Coriander, cumin, rock salt, and turmeric.

Disinfectant: (Sanskrit- Aguntaka-roganashaka) Destroys disease germs and noxious properties of fermentation; These herbs destroy pathogenic microbes (that cause communicable diseases). Examples: Apamarga, arka, gudachi, katuka, sandalwood.

Diuretic: (Sanskrit- Mutrala Karma or Mutra-virehana) Promotes the production and secretion of urine. Examples: Parsley., apamarga, ashwagandha, barberry, cardamom, cinnamon, ginger, gotu kola, gokshura, gudachi, licorice, and sandalwood.

Emetic: (Sanskrit- Vamakartya) Causes vomiting. There are three types of emetics- central, local and general. Central emetics (e.g., chamomile) act through the vomiting center of the brain. Local emetics irritate the nerves of the gastric mucus membrane (e.g., mustard). General emetics act through the blood on the vomiting center . Examples of herbs with emetic action include pippali, rock salt, vacha, ipecac, lobelia, apamarga, arka, chakramarda, chitrak and licorice.

Emmenagogue: (Sanskrit- Rajastha-paniya or Rakta- bhisarana) Herb that brings on menstruation. Herbalists also believe that these herbs clear blood congestion, blood clot; build the blood; moisten female reproductive organs; counteract aging and poor nutrition. Examples are: camomile, aloe, angelica, hibiscus, jasmine, peony, rose, and saffron.

Emollient: (Sanskrit- Snehopaga) A substance that is usually used externally to soften and soothe the skin. Examples: oils, honey, bread or bran poultice, carrots, turnips.

Expectorant: (Sanskrit- Kasa-Svasahara) Promotes the thinning and ejection of mucus or exudate from the lungs, bronchi, and trachea; sometimes the meaning is extended to all remedies that quiet a cough. Examples: ginger, licorice, calamus, cardamom, cinnamon, cloves, sage, eucalyptus, thyme, wild cherry.

Galactogogue: (Sanskrit- Stanya-janana) Increases breast milk secretion. Examples: Cumin, fennel, musta, pippali.

Germicide: Destroys germs and worms. (see disinfectant.)

Hepatic: Promotes the well-being of the liver and increases the secretion of bile. Example: golden seal.

Hypnotic: Tends to produce sleep.

Laxative: (Sanskrit- S- Svalpabhedana or Virechanlya) Herb that acts to promote evacuation of the bowels; a gentle cathartic. Examples: castor oil, flax seed, psyllium, rhubarb, senna.

Narcotic: An addicting substance that reduces pain and produces sleep.

Nervine: A substance that calms and soothes the nerves and reduces tension and anxiety. Examples: ashwagandha, bala, gudmar.

Poultice: Plant material that is prepared in a special way and applied to the surface of the body as a remedy for certain disorders.

Purgative: (Sanskrit- Virechanlya) A substance that promotes the vigorous evacuation of the bowels. Usually used to relieve severe constipation. Examples: Aloe, Epsom salt, licorice, rhubarb, safflower, senna.

Refrigerant: (Sanskrit- Dahanashaka) Relieves fever and thirst. A cooling remedy. Lowers body temperature. Examples: Aloe, coriander, ginger, hibiscus, orange, lemon, licorice, sandalwood.

Relaxant: Tends to relax and relieve tension, especially muscular tension.

Sedative: Herb that allays excitement, induces relaxation, and is conducive to sleep.

Soporific: Herbs that help to produce sleep.

Stimulant: (Sanskrit- Agni-sthapaniya or Dipana) Herb that increases the activity or efficiency of a system or organ; acts more rapidly than a tonic. Examples: cayenne, camphor,ephedra, barberry extract, yellow thistle juice, sandalwood, gotu kola, guggul, myrrh.

Stomachic: (Sanskrit- Kshudha-vardhaniya) Herbs that give strength and tone to the stomach, stimulate digestion, and improve the appetite. Examples: Amalaki, bilwa, black pepper, cardamom, cedar, chitrak, cumin, ginger, licorice, turmeric.

Sudorific: Herbs that cause heavy perspiration.

Tincture: A solution of the active principal of an herb in alcohol.

Tonic: Herbs that restore and strengthen the entire system. Produces and restores normal tone. A general tonic would be one that braces up the whole system. Example: Aloe, barberry, chirayata, guduchi, katuka, gentian, goldenseal.

Profiles of Commonly used Herbs

Alfalfa is an herb, a food, and the source of a nutritional green-food concentrate. Alfalfa is a perennial (Medicago sativa) of the pea family, widely grown as a hay feed for livestock. The Arabs considered alfalfa so nutritious that they named it the "father of all foods." In most forms it is rich in chlorophyll, beta-carotene, vitamins B6, C, and E, and calcium. As an herbal preparation, it is traditionally used as a diuretic, an arthritis remedy, and an aid to weight gain. Studies indicate it lowers blood cholesterol levels and may help prevent heart disease and possibly strokes. It is also used in sprouted form, but the leaves are more medicinal, and raw sprouts as well as seeds contain natural toxins that are potentially damaging to human health if eaten. Alfalfa's various forms include dried leaves, tablets, capsules, concentrated drops, tinctures, and extracts.

Aloe Vera preparations are derived from the leaf gel and juice of a cactus-like subgroup of the lily family with some three hundred species, including Aloe vera. The transparent get from the inner leaf is applied externally to treat burns, wounds, frostbite, and skin irritations. Studies confirm antibacterial, burn-soothing, and wound-healing effects. The gel is a common ingredient in first-aid skin creams, shampoos, and natural and conventional body care products. The plant's juice, or latex, is used to make herbal remedies to be taken internally, principally as a potent laxative. (Most herbalists recommend milder herbal laxatives such as cascara sagrada.) Studies have shown that a derivative of aloe (called Acemannan) has antitumor effects in animals and stimulates immune cells (principally macrophages) to produce cancer-fighting substances. Aloe comes in liquid, tablets, and capsules.

Angelica preparations are derived from the leaves, roots, or seeds of a tall, celery-like plant (Angelica archangelica) in the parsley family. Angelica is taken to alleviate respiratory complaints including those related to colds and flu, as well as digestive problems. Studies confirm that it has chemical compounds that relax the windpipe and intestines and thus may be beneficial for bronchitis, asthma, indigestion, and heartburn. The roots are sold dried, since the fresh root is poisonous. It's also sold in capsules, concentrated drops, extracts, and tinctures. (See Dang-gui.)

Bilberry preparations are derived from the leaves and berrylike fruit of a common European shrub (Vaccinium myrtillu) similar to the blueberry. A folk remedy for better eyesight, it gained attention when British pilots during World War II reportedly ate bilberry jam before night missions. Scientific studies confirm a positive effect on vision due to the berry's flavonoid compounds, the anthocyanoside, that can cause biochemical reactions in the eye. Bilberry may prevent acute glaucoma attacks or play a role in the treatment of chronic glaucoma. It may also play a role in relieving menstrual problems; studies have found it helps to relax smooth muscles like those found in the uterine wall.

Black cohosh preparations are derived from the dark root of a plant (Cimicifuga racemosa) also known as black snakeroot, native to North America. It is a popular Native American and folk remedy for female ailments and menstrual cramps, as well as for fatigue, anxiety, and respiratory conditions such as bronchitis. Black cohosh is also widely used in Germany for discomfort from menopause. It may have uses as a sedative and anti-inflammatory, and can lower blood pressure and possibly help control diabetes. This herb promotes menstruation, so it should be avoided during pregnancy. It has other potential side effects as well and is often recommended to be used

Burdock root (Arctium lappa) is an alterative, diaphoretic, and diuretic that is used traditionally to cleanse the blood and heal the kidneys and liver. It is one of the best blood purifiers known to traditional medicine. When taken as a tea, burdock root can also help to reduce cravings and hunger, thus assisting in weight loss. Burdock root can be eaten as food. As a dried herb, it is commonly used as a standard decoction. (To make decoction: Bring water to a boil, pour in about an ounce of dried burdock root, gently simmer for ten to twenty minutes, and allow to cool. Drink between meals.)

Calendula is a versatile and popular topical herb derived from marigold (Caledula officinalis) flowers. It has been traditionally used to treat small cuts and abrasions, inflammations, skin irritations, bruises, strains and sprains, minor burns and scalds, and hemorrhoids. It also fights bacterial, viral, and even fungal infections such as athlete's foot. Calendula a is an ingredient in many herbal combination remedies for wounds, burns, and rashes and is used to make homeopathic calendula and an essential oil. It is sold in various forms including dried, juice, concentrated drops, tinctures, and extracts.

Cascara sagrada is derived from the dried, aged bark of a small tree (Rhamnus purshiana) and is taken mainly -,is a laxative. The plant is related to buckthorn but has a much milder laxative action and causes fewer side effects. Cascara sagrada stimulates contractions in the upper intestines and also restores tone to the colon. It is included in the U.S. Pharmacopoeia and is used in many OTC laxatives. It is better for chronic constipation than stronger herbs like buckthorn, but like any herb, is not a long-term remedy for constipation. Cascara sagrada is an ingredient in the Hoxsey Cancer Formula. It is sold dried and as tablets, capsules, and concentrated drops. (See Buckthorn.)

Cayenne, also known as red pepper, is both ail herb and a spice obtained from the dried, ground fruit of various hot chili peppers (Capsicum frutescens) containing capsaicin, a compound that reduces pain and inflammation, probably by blocking the activity in the body of substance P, a compound needed for transmitting pain impulses. Capsaicin is an ingredient in some prescription skin creams. Drops of cayenne concentrate arc used to relieve toothache (though sonic will find it unpleasantly hot) and as a liniment to soothe sore muscles. Capsaicin is also used topically to stop bleeding and is taken internally to stimulate circulation or induce sweating to break a fever. Sonic herbalists use it to treat colds and infectious diarrhea. In the Far East it is a popular "crisis herb" for its heating and stimulating effects on the kidneys, lungs, stomach, and heart. It is also widely used as a spicy seasoning. It is sold in the form of capsules, concentrated drops, and tinctures.

Chamomile is an ancient and widely used herb made from the flowers of either of two annual plants (German chamomile, or Matricaria chamomilla, and Roman chamomile, or Anthemis nobilis). Taken as a tea, it has long been used to treat anxiety, insomnia, and digestive problems. Many people also apply it topically to cuts and scrapes, sore muscles, rashes, and burns. Chamomile is the source for a distinctive blue essential oil that is anti-inflammatory, analgesic, and antiseptic. Studies indicate the herb is effective at reducing fever, healing wounds, inducing sleep, and reducing the time it takes burns to heal. It seems to improve tissue regeneration and stimulate the immune-boosting activity of white blood cells. Chamomile is nontoxic and gentle enough for use on children. It's sold in various forms, including dried, teas, tablets, capsules, concentrated drops, tincturcs, and extracts.

Chaparral preparations are derived from the flowers, leaflets, and twigs of a woody, long-living shrub (Larrea tridentata, L. divaricata) of the American Southwest. Among its medically active compounds is a chemical with antibacterial action that can prevent infections when applied to wounds or can assist in clearing poor skin conditions. In the mouth, chaparral helps prevent tooth decay, mouth odor, and gum disease. Taken internally, it is a popular folk treatment for cancer; some studies confirm it may have antitumor effects. It also has potential anti-inflammatory and antioxidant properties, which may be useful in treating arthritis and helping retard aging. Chaparral was recently removed from the market by most herbal manufacturers after it was tied to five cases of acute toxic hepatitis, causing the FDA to issue a warning about it.

Chickweed (Stellaria media) has antipyretic, demulcent, and alterative properties. It is used traditionally to treat fevers, inflammation, bronchitis, pleurisy, coughs, colds, and hoarseness. It can be applied externally as a poultice to treat skin diseases. As a tea, it is effective in curbing cravings, assisting digestion, and promoting weight reduction.

Cinnamon, a common spice, has been found to triple insulin's ability to metabolize blood sugar, or glucose, according to research conducted at the Human Nutrition Research Center at Tufts University. Because of this ability, cinnamon protects against diabetes, reduces hunger, and helps control sugar cravings, thus making it easier to control weight.

Clove (Syzygiun aromaticum) contains a compound that has been shown to induce macrophages, a type Of immune cell, to target and destroy immature cancer cells more rapidly. On the other hand, clove is particularly unhealthful when consumed as an extract or in clove cigarettes. It can cause toxic reactions in the lungs, which have resulted in death when taken in high doses.

Comfrey is a popular folk herb derived from the roots and leaves of a plant (Symphytum officinale) of the borage family. It is also known as boneset and knitbone. It has traditionally been taken internally as a digestive aid and, more frequently, applied externally to promote the healing of wounds and broken bones. Studies have found comfrey to contain compounds such as allantoin that promote cell regeneration and help relieve inflammation resulting from bruises, sprains, insect bites, and skin conditions. Allantoin is now widely used in body care products for its skin-soothing properties. Applied topically, comfrey is easily absorbed through the skin and reaches deep tissue. Oral ingestion of comfrey is now rare, due to concerns about potential liver toxicity. The American Herbal Products Association recently placed comfrey on its restricted use list, for external use only.

(comfrey is frequently combined with calendula, witch hazel, St. John's wort, arnica, and other herbs in salves and ointments. It is available fresh and dried and in concentrated drops, tinctures, and extracts.

Dandelion is a bitter but nutritious herb prepared from the roots, leaves, and other parts of the well-known, widely distributed, yellow-flowered weed (Taraxacum officinale). It is also known (revealingly) as piss-in-bed. Traditionally it has been used as a digestive tonic, blood cleanser, mild diuretic and laxative, and weight loss aid. The fresh leaves are high ' in nutrients including beta-carotene, vitamin C, and potassium. As an herb, dandelion is also taken to relieve inflammation of the liver and gallbladder, congestive jaundice, skin diseases, and PMS. It may be useful to lower blood cholesterol levels, reduce high blood pressure, and prevent heart disease. Dandelion is safe and nontoxic. It is sold as tablets, capsules, concentrated drops, tinctures, and extracts.

Dong-quai, a favorite Chinese herb for women, is derived from the root of Chinese angelica (Angelica sinensis). It is also called dang-qui, dong quai, and tang kuei. It is used similarly to American and European angelica, and has long been prescribed by traditional Chinese and Indian herbalists to harmonize vital energy and nourish blood. Dang-gui is widely taken in the West for gynecological problems and to regulate hormones, alleviate menstrual cramps, and end PMS distress. It has been extensively studied in China and found to nourish the reproductive system, enhance immunity, lower blood pressure, reduce pain, and improve circulation. Dang-gui is often taken as a daily tonic by women entering menopause or before menstruation. It should be avoided during pregnancy. It comes dried and as tablets, capsules, concentrated drops, tinctures, and extracts.

Echinacea is an increasingly popular European and North American herb derived from the roots and other parts of the purple coneflower (Echinacea angustifolia, E. purpurea). It is a versatile herb used to treat a variety of injuries and illnesses. It is applied externally to cuts, bites, and stings to help promote healing, regenerate healthy cells, reduce inflammation, and maintain the structure of connective tissue. Taken internally, echinacea helps to fight bacterial and viral infections, boost the immune system, lower fever, and calm allergic reactions. Echinacea has been shown to stimulate proliferation of CD4 cells, the immune cell that is destroyed by HIV and AIDS. The herb may work best when given in small doses over a short period of time, perhaps once or twice a day over one to three days. At that point, it may be preferable to allow the herb to do its work without giving any more doses. It is nontoxic and can be taken internally in relatively large quantities (two to three dropperfuls of the tincture daily as a general immune stimulant, taken for up to a week). It is found in the form of salves, lotions, tablets, capsules, concentrated drops, tinctures, and extracts.

Eyebright preparations are derived from a northern plant (Euphrasia officinalis) with somewhat eye-shaped flowers. It has traditionally been used to make an eyewash for inflammations and other eye problems and is also taken internally for nasal congestion and coughs. Studies reveal that it contains compounds that are mildly astringent and anti-inflammatory. It is often combined with other herbs such as goldenseal, echinacea, and fennel seeds to relieve redness, swelling, and irritation of the eye. Eyebright is the source of the homeopathic remedy Euphrasia. It comes in capsules, concentrated drops, tinctures, and extracts.

Fennel preparations are produced from the seeds of a tall, stalky plant (Foeniculum vulgare) native to the Mediterranean. Fennel is primarily used as a digestive aid and to help expel gas. It is also used to treat diarrhea and infant colic. Women use it to stimulate milk flow, promote menstruation, and relieve menopausal ailments, although pregnant women should avoid it. As a tea it can be applied with an eyedropper to soothe the eyes. Aromatherapists use the essential oil medicinally, and the food industry uses it extensively as a flavoring. It is available dried and in capsules, concentrated drops, tinctures, extracts, and essential oils.

Feverfew preparations are derived from the leaves and flowers of a bushy perennial (Tanacetum parthenium) and used chiefly as a remedy for migraine headaches. Clinical trials in Britain indicate that a dosage of 50 to 100 mg daily of the dried leaves effectively prevents or significantly decreases the severity of migraine attacks for many people. Herbalists also use feverfew for its anti-inflammatory properties in the treatment of arthritis, as an antispasmodic to relieve menstrual cramps, and (as its name implies) a febrifuge. It is sold dried and in capsules, concentrated drops, tinctures, and extracts.

Garlic is an almost universally grown food and medicinal herb derived from bulbs that form on the stem of a member (Allium sativum) of the huge plant family that includes onions and leeks. As a food, it is a rich Source of protein, vitamins A, B complex, and (, and various trace minerals. Garlic has a history of medicinal use that dates back at least six thousand years. It is the basis for a seemingly endless array of folk remedies for everything from insect bites to fever. Researchers have discovered more than two hundred compounds in garlic, and scientific validation is growing for its use ill the treatment of heart disease, since it can lower both cholesterol levels and blood pressure. It is a natural antibiotic, antifungal, and antiviral that can be used internally and externally to treat food poisoning, skin conditions, and hemorrhoids. It also helps trap toxic lead and mercury in the body and remove them. Garlic is an effective antioxidant that studies show may reduce the risk of stomach cancer. It is widely used in cooking, though heat inactivates its enzymes and significantly reduces its medicinal effects. Garlic is available fresh 01- juiced as well as in tablets, capsules, concentrated drops, tinctures, and extracts.

Ginger is derived from the underground stem and root of a tropical plant (Zingiber officinale) native to the Far East. It has been used since ancient times by the Greeks, Chinese, and others as a medicine and flavoring. Ginger is widely taken today for its calling effect on the digestive system and is the premier natural remedy for nausea from morning sickness, upset stomach, and motion sickness. It helps expel gas from the intestines and relaxes and soothes the intestinal tract. Ginger has been shown to reduce the production of prostaglandins that cause inflammation, especially in people with arthritis. Such swelling, of course, is one of the factors that cause and exacerbate arthritis pain. Researchers have found that ginger also inhibits platelet aggregation, which means it prevents the blood from sludging, one of the factors that give rise to heart attacks and strokes. Ginger may also lower blood cholesterol levels. It is nontoxic and safe to take in large doses. It comes fresh or dried and in tablets, capsules, concentrated drops, tinctures, and extracts.

Ginkgo preparations are derived from the fan-shaped leaves of one of the world's most ancient tree species (Ginko biloba). It has been used by the Chinese for thousands of years to treat asthma, allergies, and coughs. Currently it is gaining popularity for its reputed ability to improve brain function and boost memory and alertness. Researchers say that it stimulates circulation in the brain and ears and thus may help prevent dizziness, hearing loss, tinnitus, stroke, and depression. Ginkgo acts as an antioxidant. Studies indicate it has potential use in the treatment of impotence, varicose veins, and Alzheimer's disease. Extracts are often standardized to contain 24 percent ginkgo heterosides. it comes in tablets, capsules, concentrated drops, tinctures, and extracts.

Ginseng is a human-shaped root that is one of the most popular healing herbs of the East and West. It includes species from Asia (Panax ginseng, usually called Chinese or Korean ginseng) and North America (P. quinquefolius, called American ginseng). Siberian ginseng, or eleuthero, is also from the ginseng family and has similar effects and uses. Ginseng is commonly used as an adaptogen, meaning it normalizes physical functioning regardless of direction (for example, it will lower high blood pressure, but raise low blood pressure). It is also typically taken to lessen the effects of stress, improve performance, boost energy levels, enhance memory, and stimulate immunity. One study showed that two polysaccharides that could be isolated from ginseng stimulated the proliferation of CD4 cells in response to a disease-causing agent. Ginseng protects cells from damage by radiation and toxic substances. It is not as stimulating as herbs containing caffeine or ephedrine, but may be too strong for some people and should be used in moderation. It is sold as a whole root or powder and in capsules, tablets, tea bags, tinctures, and extracts. (See Siberian ginseng.)

Goldenseal preparations are derived from the yellow root of a small perennial plant (Hydrastis canadensis) native to eastern North America. One of the most widely used herbs, with both internal and external applications, it is taken orally to alleviate colds, fevers, digestive ailments, and infectious diarrhea, and to stimulate the immune system. Studies confirm that its compound berberine has pharmacological powers, notably the abilities to fight bacteria and to Stimulate immunity. Goldenseal reduces excessive menstrual flow. Topically, it is used for its anti-inflammatory and antiseptic actions and is widely recommended by herbalists to clean Wounds, alleviate skin infections or sores (including ringworm, athlete's foot, and itching), and reduce hemorrhoids. It shouldn't be taken long-term in large amounts or by pregnant women or people with high blood pressure. It is often expensive and sometimes adulterated. It is sold as a powder and in capsules, concentrated drops, and extracts.

Gotu kola is a principally Asian plant (Hydrocotyle asiatica, Centella asiatica). It should not be confused with kola, an unrelated, caffeine-containing herb. For thousands of years gotu kola has been a popular remedy in India and Pakistan, where it has a reputation for promoting longevity and is being investigated for use against leprosy and tuberculosis. In the West, it is used mainly as a tonic to increase energy and endurance, improve memory and mental stamina, and alleviate depression and anxiety. It boosts circulation in the legs and is an effective remedy for varicose veins. (gotu kola also has important uses externally as a wound healer, burn remedy, and psoriasis treatment. Large doses taken internally may have a sedating effect. It is sold dried and in capsules, concentrated drops, tinctures, and extracts.

Green tea, taken either in capsule form or as a beverage (both available in natural foods stores), provides numerous health benefits. Green tea contains chemical compounds called polyphenols (not present in the more common black teas), which act as powerful antioxidants. Studies show that people who drink approximately five cups of green tea a day (which contains about half the caffeine of coffee) or who take 500 mg a day of the caffeine-free capsules, have a lower risk of incurring cancer, suffering heart attacks and strokes, and contracting gum disease and cavities. Human population studies and animal research have shown a strong correlation between green tea consumption and reduced risk of certain cancers, especially esophageal cancer. The polyphenols in green tea also attack the bacteria that cause bad breath.

Hawthorn preparations are derived from the flowers, leaves, or berries of a thorny shrub (Crataegus oxyacantha) native to Europe. It enjoys a long history of use as a heart tonic, and studies have confirmed that the plant is a rich source of bioflavonoids and other chemical compounds that affect heart function. Hawthorn is an effective antioxidant. It can reduce blood pressure and prevent palpitations, arrhythmias, and atherosclerosis. Hawthorn helps stabilize collagen, the protein normally found in joints that is destroyed during inflammation, and thus may be useful against arthritis. Hawthorn is best taken over a prolonged period. It is sold as dried berries, capsules, tinctures, and extracts.

Hops is derived from the cone-like fruits of a climbing plant (Humulus lupulus) best known for giving beer its bitter flavor. It is a digestive stimulant that is particularly effective for digestive complaints caused by anxiety. It is also a mild sedative and a diuretic. It is sold dried and as concentrated drops, tinctures, and extracts.

Kelp is a nutrient-dense brown sea vegetable that is among the richest sources of the element iodine, which is needed by thyroid hormones to help regulate the body's growth and development. Iodine can also protect cells from damage by radioactive substances and heavy metals. As a food, kelp is usually eaten in small quantities; it is also used as a condiment and nutritional supplement. There are some potential adverse effects from long-term overuse. it is sold dried or as a liquid, powder, or tablets.

Lemon balm preparations are derived from the aromatic leaves of a perennial mint plant (Melissa officinalis). Also known as balm, bee balm, and sweet balm, it has traditionally been used to relieve nervousness and anxiety or to induce sweating. Studies confirm that it relaxes the nervous system and is an effective though mild herbal sedative. Herbalists recommend, it to alleviate headaches, anxiety, and depression that are caused by nervous problems. It also improves digestion. Lemon balm is used topically as a wound healer. It has been found to have antibacterial, antiviral, and analgesic properties. Lemon balm is among the gentlest of the calming herbs, which include skullcap, valerian, hops, and passionflower. It is available dried and as concentrated drops, tinctures, and extracts.

Licorice is an herb prepared from the roots of an Oriental and European perennial (Glycyrrhiza globra) of the pea family. Licorice has long been used by traditional Chinese, Greek, and European herbalists as a general tonic and for respiratory problems such as asthma, coughs, and bronchitis. Studies have confirmed potential uses to relieve coughs, treat ulcers, alleviate arthritis, and control liver conditions such as hepatitis and cirrhosis. The herb's natural sweetness makes it a favorite flavor for herbal combination products as well as for candies and other foods. Overuse of extracts may cause adverse health effects related to salt and water retention. Retailers sell licorice in powders, capsules, concentrated drops, tinctures, and extracts.

Milk thistle is a traditional liver remedy prepared from the seeds of a thorny, weed-like plant (Cardus marianum). It is often taken in the form of silymarin, a standardized extract of a complex compound found in the seeds. Studies confirm that silymarin helps liver cells regenerate and stabilizes liver cell membranes. It also boosts the organ's ability to filter blood and prevents liver damage from toxins including solvents, alcohol, drugs, most pesticides and herbicides, and bacteria] compounds like those associated with food poisoning. Milk thistle may help treat cirrhosis, hepatitis, and other liver diseases. It is often taken regularly as a preventive and after exposure to a toxin. It comes in capsules, concentrated herbal drops, and extracts.

Mint, such as spearmint and peppermint, is high in calcium, vitamins A and C, and riboflavin. Peppermint is useful for allaying insomnia, upset stomachs, and nervous tension. Mint has also been shown to increase the number of phagocyte cells) which are capable of destroying pathogens, bacteria, and cancer cells. Mints are available in dried herb form and as oils and extracts.

Mullein preparations are derived from the leaves, roots, or flowers of a tall, spike-like plant (Verbascum thapsus) used to make traditional respiratory remedies. Chemical analysis confirms that mullein contains mucilage, a substance that relieves coughs and soothes sore throats by absorbing water in the windpipe and becoming slippery. Mullein also acts as an expectorant by bringing up mucus. Herbalists use a mullein flower oil infusion (not the essential oil) as drops to relieve earaches. Mullein is sold dried or as concentrated drops, tinctures, extracts, oils, and essential oils.

Nettle supplements are derived from the upper leaves and steins of a stinging, weed-like plant (Urtica dioica, U. urens) found around the world. It is also known as stinging nettle. As a healing herb, it is taken as a euphoria, and it can relieve headaches or general tonic and to relieve hay fever, asthma, high blood pressure, PMS, and eczema. Nettle has astringent and diuretic properties. Applied externally by flailing a joint with the stinging plant ("urtication"), it may help relieve the paiii of artliritis and gout. Nettles arc also taken as a "super-food" rich in vitamins C and E and minerals Such as calcium, magnesium, iron, silica, and potassium, which are important for healing broken bones, muscle strains, and tendon injuries. You can sprinkle dried nettles on salads, soups, and vegetables. It is sold dried and freeze-dried and in capsules, tinctures, concentrated drops, and extracts.

Passionflower preparations are made from the leaves of a climbing vine (Passiflora incarnata). Passionflower has traditionally been used as a sedative and analgesic. It can help induce a contemplative state or mild muscle spasms from nervous tension. Passionflower is gentle enough for children who are overly nervous and for the elderly suffering from insomnia. It is also an antispasmodic sometimes recommended as a digestive aid and menstrual reliever. It is not an aphrodisiac, despite its name, which derives from the plant's supposed resemblance to the crown of thorns in the Biblical Passion. It should be avoided by pregnant women and shouldn't be taken in large amounts. It is sold dried and in concentrated drops, tinctures, and extracts.

Pau d'arco preparations derive from the inner bark of a tail, flowering tree (Tabebuia avellanedae, T. impetiginosa) native to Brazil. The herb, also known as lapacho and taheebo, has been used for centuries in South America to heal wounds and treat snakebites. Its popularity is spreading among herbalists in the United States and Europe due to its broad clinical applications, including antibacterial, antiviral, and anti-inflammatory properties. The tea and extract can be taken orally or applied topically for bites and stings, infections, and inflammations. It comes as dried, shredded bark or as capsules and liquid extracts (often standardized for lapachol content).

Red raspberry is prepared from the leaves and berries of a prickly bush (Rubus idaeus). It has traditionally been used as a woman's herb to control morning sickness during pregnancy and to case the pain of mensturation and childbirth. It has also long been used as a remedy for childhood diarrhea. Studies confirm that it helps relax the uterus and contains astringent compounds that can treat diarrhea. It is sold dried and in capsules, concentrated drops, tinctures, and extracts.

Rosemary is a strong-smelling herb and essential oil made from the thin leaves of a small evergreen shrub (Rosmarinus officinalis). It has long been a popular cooking herb and an ingredient in a stimulating tonic wine said to have a positive effect on the nervous and circulatory systems. Rosemary is used to treat chronic circulatory weakness, including low blood pressure. It is also an appetite stimulator, digestive aid, and antioxidant. It is applied topically to soothe sprains and bruises and heal wounds. A few drops of the essential oil put in the bath act as a relaxant. Taken internally, the essential oil may induce menses and thus should be avoided by pregnant women. Rosemary comes dried and in tinctures, concentrated drops, and essential oils.

St. John's wort preparations are derived from the leaves and flowers of a common North American and European perennial (Hypericum perforatum) that has been used since antiquity as a topical wound healer. Studies have identified biologically active compounds with potential wound-healing, immune-boosting, and antibiotic properties. It has also traditionally been taken internally for depression, insomnia, and anxiety. Researchers confirm that St. John's wort acts like the antidepressive drugs known as MAO inhibitors to elevate mood. Homeopaths use the plant to make the widely used Hypericum preparations. It is usually sold dried and in concentrated drops, tinctures, and extracts.

Senna is derived from the leaflets and seed pods of a small shrub (Cassia angustifolia) grown in India. An ingredient in conventional laxatives, it is taken for its powerful effects on constipation. Herbalists often combine it with ginger or other herbs to reduce its side effects, which i-nay include sudden, sharp bowel pains. Most herbalists recommend trying milder laxatives like cascara sagrada first. Senna should be avoided by pregnant women and should not be taken for an extended time. It comes in capsules, tinctures, and extracts.

Shepherd's purse preparations are derived from the flowering tops of a common North American weed (Capsella bursa pastoris) of the mustard family. Its name comes from its distinctive, purse-shaped seed pods. Shepherds purse has been used since ancient times to stop bleeding, both internal (menstrual bleeding, for instance) and external (cuts, scrapes, and nosebleeds). Chemical analysis confirms that it contains tyramines and other chemicals that promote blood coagulation and constrict blood vessels. It also has compounds (choline and acetylcholine) that reduce blood pressure. Shepherd's purse may trigger labor during pregnancy. It is available dried and in capsules, concentrated drops, tinctures, and extracts.

Slippery elm preparations are derived from the ground inner I)ark of a tree (Ulmus rubra, U. fulva) recently ravaged in the United States by Dutch elm disease. It has been a popular folk medicine, healing food, and digestive tonic for thousands of years. Today it is most widely used in lozenges for symptomatic relief of sore throats, coughs, and colds. As a paste it can be used externally to soothe and heal minor skin injuries, rashes, and irritations - even the FDA calls it an excellent demulcent, or soothing agent. Slippery elm can be mixed with water or milk to make a food that, because it is nutritious and easily assimilated) is often recommended for those recovering from illness. It is sold in powders, lozenges, tablets, and extracts.

Valerian is an "herbal Valium" prepared from the root of a European plant (Valeriana officinalis) now spread throughout the northeastern United States. Valerian is taken to provide temporary relief from anxiety and to prevent insomnia. It can also help relieve headaches, stomach and menstrual cramps, and constipation or indigestion from nervous tension. Studies have found it is as effective as some barbiturates for reducing the time needed to fall asleep, though it is stimulating instead of calming to some people. It is safe when taken in moderate doses (a gram of the powder, a teaspoon of the tincture, or 250 nig of the liquid or solid extract) but should not be used for an extended period of time. Valerian is sold dried and in tablets, capsules, concentrated drops, tinctures, and extracts.

Vitex, well known in Europe as "the women's herb," is derived from the berries of a Mediterranean plant (Vitex agnuscastus). The herb is also known as chaste tree, chasteberry, and agnus castus. In the Middle Ages, vitex was thought to have an antiaphrodisiac effect. Today it is used principally to treat women's conditions such as PMS, menopausal discomfort, fibroids, and excessive menstrual bleeding. It works to balance hormones by strengthening the sexual organs and glands. Vitex also stimulates the flow of breast milk and may clear acne during puberty. It is safe for use over an extended period of time. It comes in tablets, capsules, concentrated drops, tinctures, and extracts.

White willow preparations are made from the bark of a tree (Salix alba) and are used to relieve pain and reduce fever. Like the herb meadowsweet (Filipendula ulmaria), white willow bark is a natural source of salicum, a chemical relative of the synthetic salicylic acid used to make aspirin (acetylsalicylic acid). Some willow-based aspirin substitutes are standardized for the salicin content. Because of the risk of Reye's syndrome, white willow preparations shouldn't be given to children who have fevers that may be due to certain viral illnesses. The herb comes fresh and dried, and in tablets, concentrated drops, tinctures, and extracts.

Witch hazel is a widely used medicinal herb derived from the leaves and bark of a North American shrub or small tree (Hamamelis virginiana). It is used as a liniment even by medical doctors and is available in conventional pharmacies. It has well-established astringent properties that reduce the pain and swelling of hemorrhoids, varicose veins, insect bites, and bruises. It is also an effective styptic that can stop the bleeding from small cuts such as shaving nicks. Witch hazel is a component in some cosmetics. Witch hazel is mild enough to be applied directly to the skin and is a popular ingredient in herbal skin salves. It comes in concentrated drops, tinctures, and extracts.

Yarrow preparations are derived from the leaves, stems, and flower tops of a common North American weed (Achillea millefolium). It is traditionally used to make topical preparations to stem bleeding and promote the healing of wounds. It has astringent and antiseptic properties, and studies have identified more than a hundred biologically active compounds in its tissues. Today, yarrow is principally used externally on burns, cuts, bruises, and hemorrhoids. It is also used internally to relieve cramps, menstrual bleeding, and fevers, and to treat colds and flu. It is sold fresh and dried and in concentrated drops, tinctures, and extracts.

Yellow dock (also known as curly dock) preparations are derived from the leaves and roots of a widespread weed (Rumex crispus) of the buckwheat family. It has traditionally been used as a blood tonic and liver rejuvenator and is applied topically to treat chronic skin sores and ringworm. In low doses, it is a gentle laxative. Large doses can cause nausea. It comes in capsules, concentrated drops, tinctures, and extracts.

Yohimbe is an aphrodisiac derived from the bark of the yohimbe tree (Corynanthe yohimbe), an evergreen indigenous to West Africa. Studies demonstrate its aphrodisiac effects on men. Yohimbe can cause erectile stimulation of the penis and help in the treatment of male impotence. The compound yohimbine hydrochloride is the active ingredient in some prescription drugs (Actibine, Aphrodyne, Yohimex) for types of male impotence. The herb may also elevate mood and may be a weight loss aid. According to FDA regulations, it cannot be promoted in herbal form as an aphrodisiac.

Herbal Reference Chart

Common uses and Actions of Chinese, Native American, and Western herbs.

Common Name	**Actions**	**Uses**	**Combine With**
Arnica Flowers	Topical Bruises and Sprains	Strains, sprains, over- exertion	Comfrey Root
Astragalus	Enhances the immune system and restores peripheral circulation	Cold & Flu	Pau D Arco, Garlic, Schisandra, Echinacea
Bilberry	Antioxidant, Stabilizes Collagen, Vascular Disorders	Eye disorders such as night blindness	Eyebright, Rosehips
Boswellia	Anti-inflammatory, Sedative	Arthritis, sports Injuries	Quercetin
Burdock Root	Blood Cleanser	Skin Conditions and Boils	Yellow Dock, Milk Thistle
Calendula	Anti-Inflammatory	Burns, Wounds, Abscesses	Aloe Vera, Pau D' Arco
Chamomile	Carminative, Digestive Aid	Relaxation, Sleep	Valerian, Kava, Passion Flower
Chaste Berry	PMS, Menopause	Normalizes pituitary function	Red Raspberry, Dong Quai
Coltsfoot	Anti-spasmodic	Bronchitis, Asthma, Coughs	Horehound, Echinacea

Cranberry	Diuretic	Kidney, Bladder	Uva Ursi, Cornsilk
Echinacea	Anti-viral, Antiseptic, Immune Stimulant	Cold & Flu Infections	Goldenseal, Pau D Arco Ginseng, Garlic
Feverfew	Anti-inflammatory	Migraines, Headaches	Valerian
Garlic	Antibiotic, Antiseptic, Antiviral	Cold & Flu	Echinacea, Goldenseal, Astragulas
Ginger Root	Digestive Aid, Reduces Nausea	Morning Sickness	Peppermint
Ginkgo Biloba	Cerebral Circulation	Mental Clarity, Alertness	Gotu Kola
Green Tea	Antioxidant	Energy	Astragulas
Gotu Kola	Endurance	Mental Stamina, Improves Memory	Ginseng
Hawthorn	Dilates blood Vessels	Heart	Ginseng
Hops	Sedative, Reduces Muscle Spasm	Relaxation, Sleep Aid	Valerian, Kava
Horehound	Expectorant	Respiratory Congestion	Coltsfoot

Kava	Sedative	Stress Anxiety	Valerian
Ma Huang	Vasodilator	Hay Fever	Pleurisy Root
Milk Thistle	Protects Against Toxins	Liver Detox	Burdock, Dandelion
Mullein Leaf	Expectorant	Earaches	Garlic
Nettles Leaf	Anti-histamine, Nutritive	Eczema, Hay fever, Allergies	Oregon Grape
Pau D Arco	Anti-fungal, Blood Cleanser	Candida	Grapefruit Seed Extract
Red Raspberry	Uterine Tonic	Painful Menses, Bleeding Gums	Ginger Root
Saw Palmetto	Anti-inflammatory	Prostate Problems	Pumpkin seed oil
St. Johns Wort	Anti-depressant	Depression	Kava, Valerian
Valerian	Sleep Aid	Tension, Anxiety, Insomnia, Stress	Kava
Wild Yam	Anti-spasmodic, Carminative	Ovarian & Uterine Pain	Don Quai
Yellow Dock	Mild Laxative, Blood Cleanser	Skin Disorders	Milk Thistle

Common Conditions and their Herbal Remedies

Anxiety: Valerian, Passion Flower

Arthritis: Devil's Claw, Boswellia, Evening Primrose Oil

Blood Pressure: Garlic, Hawthorn

Cholesterol (High): Garlic, Gugulipid

Circulation (Poor): Ginkgo biloba, Garlic, Cayenne, Hawthorn

Colds/Flu: Echinacea, Astragalus, Garlic, Goldenseal Root

Constipation: Aloe, Cascara sagrada, Senna, Psyllium

Coughs: Licorice, Wild Cherry Bark, Thyme

Depression (Mild): St. John's Wort, Valerian

Detoxification: Milk Thistle (Silymarin)

Digestion (Poor): Chamomile, Peppermint, Ginger

Fatigue: Panax Ginseng, Eleuthero (Siberian Ginseng)

Insomnia: Valerian, Passion Flower, Hops, Lemon Balm

Memory Loss: Ginkgo biloba

Migraine Headache: Feverfew

Menstrual Irregularities/PMS: Dong Quai, Vitex agnus-castus, Evening Primrose Oil

Nausea: Ginger, Chamomile, Peppermint

Skin Conditions: Calendula, Chamomile (topical), Tea Tree Oil (topical)

Stress/Tension: Valerian, Passion Flower, Kava Kava, Eleuthero (Siberian Ginseng)

Ulcers: Licorice, Aloe juice

Urinary Tract Problems: Cranberry, Uva Ursi

Water Retention: Uva Ursi, Dandelion Leaf

General Guidelines For Using Herbs

Herbal remedies have a long history of traditional uses, many of which are supported by scientific research and by personal experience. The remedies most often suggested by herbalists come in specific forms: teas, tinctures, capsules, herbal vinegars, salves, poultices or suppositories. Tinctures are more convenient than teas and are more potent. Capsules are widely available and convenient to take, but are not always absorbed as well as liquid preparations. First, figure out what herbs you will need. Start with high quality herbs that you have grown yourself or obtained from reliable sources.

Homemade preparations are much less costly than store-bought products. You can custom make remedies to suit your needs by mixing and matching different combinations of herbs into teas and tinctures. Start simply, using one herb at a time so you can learn the properties of that herb before you mix it with others. Follow recommended dosages and make sure you know the herbal properties of each herb. Do not mix herbal remedies and prescription drugs without professional advice.

Utensils: Use glass, enamel or stainless steel pots and pans, wooden or steel knives and spatulas and plastic, nylon or stainless steel sieves. Never use aluminum utensils; aluminum is potentially toxic and easily absorbed by herbs. A double boiler is useful for making oils, creams and salves. A good coffee bean grinder is valuable for grinding tough bark, berries and roots. Use only for herbs or your coffee will taste like herbs and your herbs like coffee. A good blender is necessary to make skin creams. You will need jars and bottles for tinctures, salves, oils and vinegars. You can recycle wide-mouth food jars and salad dressing bottles or purchase new ones. You may need to order special smaller bottles or jars with droppers for tinctures, or small glass or plastic jars for salves. All utensils should be sterilized for at least 30 minutes in a well diluted sterilizing solution. After soaking, rinse thoroughly with boiling water and dry in a hot oven or dish-washer. Proper sterilization prevents remedies, especially creams and syrups, from becoming moldy.

Herbal Teas: Infusions and Decoctions: Herbal teas require a longer steeping time than traditional green or black tea. An infusion is an herbal tea made with leaves or flowers. For a hot infusion, boiling water is poured over the tea, the cup or pot is covered and left to sit for 10-20 minutes or more, and the herb is strained out. Use cold water if the herb will deteriorate in hot water. If using cold water, 12-20 hours are required for steeping. Use clear soft or distilled water. Standard quantities are 1-2 teas. dried herb or 2-3 teas. fresh herb per cup boiling water, 3-4 times per day. A decoction is made from roots, bark, twigs or berries that usually require a more forceful treatment than leaves or flowers to extract the medicinal forces. Herbs are placed in a pan, water is added, the pan covered and simmered on very low heat, 20-30 minutes, the heat is turned off, and the herbs are left to stand another 10-20 minutes before straining. Strain through a fine-mesh strainer into a glass jar or mug. Press herbs with the back of a spoon in order to extract as much liquid as possible. For some herbs you may need to use a coffee filter to strain out fine hairs or irritating particles. In combination decoctions and infusions, first prepare the decoction with sufficient water, then turn off the heat and add the herbs to be infused.

Tinctures or Fluid Extracts: A tincture is an herbal preparation whose medicinal virtues are extracted into solution with grain alcohol, vegetable glycerine, or vinegar. Certain medicine principles are not retrieved in water alone. Alcohol (diluted 100% pure grain alcohol or vodka, which is usually 40-50% alcohol) or vinegar (unfiltered apple cider), are the best solvents. Alcohol makes a better preservative for long-term storage of extracts.

Alcohol or vinegar tinctures can be made by taking approximately 4 ounces ground dried herbs or 8 ounces of finely chopped fresh herbs, place them in a glass bottle with at least 16 ounces of alcohol or vinegar. If the herb is not completely submerged, add more alcohol or vinegar. Cap tightly, and each day for at least 10-14 days, or longer, shake vigorously. Shake more often if using dried herbs. Then extract the liquid, squeezing through cloth, canvas or muslin, or use a wine press. Place the tincture extract in dark bottles, cover tightly and store in a dark, cool place. When administering a tincture internally, you may evaporate the alcohol from the solution by putting it into hot water, or it can be taken as is. Alcohol is preferred where there are resinous or oily herb extracts, as glycerine or vinegar will not dissolve or mix completely with these. Alcohol extracts will generally last 5-10 years or more, depending upon the percentage of alcohol in the final product. Vinegar extracts will usually lasts 1-2 years.

A glycerine extract can be made by soaking 4 ozs. of ground dried herb in 12 ozs. of water (or 8 oz. fresh herb in 6 oz. water), adding 6-10 ozs. of glycerine (depending upon how long the extract needs sto be preserved). Macerate for 10 days or more; strain and bottle. You can also make a concentrated herbal tea (reduce by 1/2 or more), strain, and add 50% - 75% glycerine. Vegetable glycerine does not dissolve resinous or oily herbs, which require alcohol as a solvent. Another way is to first make a grain alcohol extract from the desired herb(s) and then remove the alcohol from the solution by low heating, adding back 50 to 75% vegetable glycerine. Glycerine extracts will last from 1 - 2 years, depending upon the amount of glycerine added as preservative.

Oils, Salves and Creams: The essential oils can be extracted from any herb. By using different herbal combinations and different oils to extract the herbal essences, you can make both strong medicinal oils and scented massage and bath oils. Olive oil is the oil of choice because it is of high quality, and has nutritious and medicinal substances of its own. It also lasts longer than other oils. You can also use almond, sunflower seed, sesame, grape seed, apricot, or other vegetable oils. When using oils, start with freshly dried herbs. If you want to use fresh, at least let them wilt overnight. Then, when you add the oil, cover with muslin to let moisture escape. There are several methods used to extract the oils: Solar Infused

Oils: Place the herbs (either dry or freshly wilted) in a quart jar. Fill the jar with the oil you have selected. There must be enough oil to completely cover the herbs, with at least 2 to 3 inches of oil above. Cover tightly. Place in a warm, sunny spot. Let sit in the sunlight at least 2 weeks. Shake daily. Strain and bottle. Oven Extracted Oils: Place the herbs in a saucepan. Cover the herbs with enough oil to completely cover the top of the herbs by at least 2-3" of oil. Place a tight-fitting lid on the pan. Turn oven on lowest temperature (generally around 150 degrees) and allow to steep for 5-10 hours; check frequently. Be sure you are not deep frying your herbs or sizzling your oil. Strain and bottle. Double Boiler Method: This is probably the most popular method because it takes the least time. Place the herbs in a double boiler. Cover with oil. Cook over boiling water (a low simmer) for several hours. The water should be boiling, not the herbs. Strain and bottle. Crock Pot Method: This is my favorite method. Set the gauge at the lowest temperature setting (80-125 degrees, no higher). Place the herbs in the pot and cover with oil. It usually takes 6-8 hours or longer at a constant temperature, to completely extract the plant properties. If you are not sure if the temperature of your crock pot is low enough, keep the pot on for an hour and cool for an hour, 6 - 8 times, until you are satisfied that the herbs are done.

Salves or Ointments: A salve is a semi-solid medicinal preparation designed for use on the skin, with protective emollient properties. Salves usually consist of a wax, herbs, and vegetable or animal fat. The oil is the solvent used to extract the herbal properties; it also provides a soothing base. The wax solidifies the salve. To each cup of infused and strained herbal oil, add one ounce of beeswax. Melt the oil and beeswax together in a double boiler. Then you can add essential oils, Vitamin A or E, or other ingredients. You may substitute coconut oil or cocoa butter for part of the oil and wax. Lanolin also makes a soothing addition to salves. If you substitute these solid ingredients you will need to reduce the amount of beeswax. Pour the liquid salve into containers while still warm. Salves are applied directly on the skin and are used for eczema, cuts, diaper rashes, scratches, wounds, burns, chapped lips, sunburn, etc.

Creams or Lotions: A cream or lotion is a light oil preparation emulsified with a medicated liquid. While similar to an ointment or salve, it has the advantage of penetrating faster and promoting healing. It allows the skin to breathe by not clogging the pores. Creams should be used sparingly and often. They quickly moisten, sooth and cool the skin in all dry, irritated or hot skin conditions. To make your cream, you'll need two kinds of ingredients: oil-based and water-based. All ingredients must be at room temperature. Put the water-based ingredients into a blender. Turn on high and slowly add the oil-based ingredients. Pour into bottles and cap. Creams and lotions will not last very long unless a preservative is added. The best natural preservatives are Vitamins C and E.

Poultice/Compress/Plaster: A poultice is a water, tincture or fresh herb-based external medication applied topically for a short time. A poultice can often be changed and renewed, so it is more versatile than a plaster. When using fine herb powder, add just use enough moisture to make a thick paste; when using the granulated form, a thick paste may be made with a mixture of water and cornmeal or flaxseed meal. If fresh green leaves are used, simply heat, bruise, and chop them up finely, and apply to the affected part. Wrap in coarse muslin, cheesecloth or wool to keep them in place. Poultices are excellent for enlarged or inflamed glands and also for eruptions, boils, carbuncles and abscesses.

A compress (also known as a fomentation) is a cloth soaked in a strong herbal tea or tincture. The main function of a cold compress is to stimulate and decongest in cold conditions such as edema, amenorrhea, constipation and scanty urination, reduce fever and inflammation, and to decongest in hot conditions such as congested head, liver or feet, and relieve tiredness due to overwork or stress on the feet, legs or hands. A warm or hot compress is used to restore strength and reduce fatigue, to relax and loosen muscle spasms, aches or pains, muscle tension, neuralgia or relieve skin rashes. Alternate hot and cold compresses can be used in first-aid and internal conditions to relieve stagnation, fluid congestion, and physical lumps and tumors. To make a compress: Fold and immerse a piece of toweling, flannel or other cloth in cold or hot herb tea, tincture or essential oil preparation of 1% dilution. Leave the compress on for two to four hours, changing if necessary.

A plaster is an herbal preparation for external application that is harder than an ointment, but soft enough to be spread on cloth and adhere to the skin when applied to the body. The consistency of a plaster will vary according to the intended purpose --those applied to the breast or stomach will be soft and yielding, while those applied to the extremities should be firm and adhesive. Plasters must always be watched so that they are not left on too long, as some types such as mustard plasters may cause blisters or burns.

Capsules and Pills: Capsules come in 0 (small) and 00 (large) sizes. To fill a capsule, take the two halves apart and push these halves into finely ground herb powder and toward each other. Small devices that help to encapsulate herbs into 50 capsules at a time are available. Capsules are a convenient way to take herbs, but the powdering process can cause loss of herb quality, and digestion is not always complete.

In one method of making an herbal pill, the herbal agent is ground into a very fine powder and mixed with a mucilage of gum Arabic, slippery elm, or a syrup which is then worked up into a pill mass. A portion is then cut off, sliced into small strips and then into smaller pill-sized pieces, which are then rolled into little round balls. In another method, the dried, powdered herbs are mixed with slippery elm or even flour, then rolled like a pie dough and passed through a large screen to make square pills. In either method, the pills are then placed in a warm place to dry thoroughly.

Liniments: Liniments can be applied by rubbing or massage, and have excellent warming effects. They stimulate, warm and relax the skin and muscles in external conditions. They relieve local tissue trauma with swelling such as sprains. They relieve burns and inflammation, and also repel insects. Liniments can be oil or water based. To make an oil-based liniment, mix herbs in oil or lard over very low heat for 4-8 hours, then strain. Use 1 pint of lard or oil for every 2 ounces of dried herbs. Alternately, soak the material for 2-3 weeks, shaking it once or twice daily. Strain and store. A water-based liniment is made exactly the same way as a tincture, except rubbing alcohol is used. If this is the case, be sure to label the bottle clearly "For external use only."

Bath/Wash: Therapeutic baths use water to which herbal teas or bundled herbs have been added. The purpose of an herbal bath is to restore and strengthen, to relax, calm and release tension, to stimulate and warm, to reduce fever in feverish conditions (cool bath), and to draw out toxins. Full Bath: A cold full body bath is taken for 1-2 mins., never longer. For those in good health, it has a reviving and stimulating effect. A warm full bath has a sedating effect. Warm full baths are mildly relaxing. They can generally treat tension and stress. Crush or chop the herbs to be used, using up to 4 ozs. Add to water and allow to steep covered for 4-5 hours. This can be used for several baths. Use 2/3-1 pint of the herb tea for each bath, or add essential oils, 5-10 drops directly in the water. The herb mix may be bound up in a muslin bag and steeped in the hot water for the entire duration of the bath. Sitzbath: Fill a bowl or bathtub with enough water to cover the hips up to the waist only. Add 1/2 pint of the herbal preparation or 5-10 drops of essential oil to the water. Cold sitzbaths should last only 1-3 minutes. They are unsurpassed for heavy menstruation and boost the immunity to help prevent colds and flues. A hot sitzbath of about 15 minutes will stimulate, relax and relieve pain. They are typically used for painful menses, hemorrhoids and constipation.

Bolus/Suppository: A suppository or bolus is an herbal preparation in the shape of a cone or cylinder, used to apply the herbal agent into the nostrils, rectum, urethra or vagina. These solid formations are introduced into the different body orifices. To make a bolus or suppository, add slippery elm or cocoa butter to powdered herbs. Add water to the combination to make a dough-like mass that is easily formed.

Shape into long pencil shaped tubes and cut into the desired size. These are easily inserted and will melt at body temperature.

Electuary: This is an herbal powder incorporated into honey or syrup to form a soft or pasty mass which can be rolled into a ball. When a child does not like to take capsules or resists drinking strong teas, you can make up an electurary by mixing herb powder with a little honey, stiffening it with a small quantity of coconut or slippery elm powder, and then have the child chew the mass. Even cayenne can be taken in this way, using peanut butter and honey as a base. Electuaries may be made from powders of barks, roots, seeds and flowers, but astringent electuaries (having pulps or fruits in them) should be prepared only in small quantities, as the medicinal virtues in these are rapidly lost and the fruit pulps are apt to ferment.

Enema: This is a way to administer copious amounts of liquid into the bowel itself, including infusions or decoctions, having a laxative or peristaltic action upon the bowels. It is also used as a means of conveying nutritive fluids into the system. There are anti-putrefaction enemas, diuretic enemas, emollient enemas, laxative enemas. If a hot or warm enema is given, then the anus will relax, causing the rectal area to discharge immediately, so a cool preparation is preferred as it will soak through the waste concentrations. Prepare an infusion or decoction with 1 1/2 teaspoons of herb to each cup of water. Use 1 1/2 cups to 1 pint solution for children. Use 1 to 3 quarts for adults.

Syrup: A syrup is a thick, sweet liquid used for irritated conditions of the throat, lungs, stomach and intestines where continuous soothing effects are needed. It coats the digestive passages. The gradual and gentle absorption of syrups is ideal for children and elderly people. Syrup is made by dissolving sugar or honey into distilled water, decoctions, infusions, or juices, and is used to suspend medicinal or flavoring agents for easy administration alone, or to combine with other preparations. To make a syrup with herbs, for every pint of double strength herbal liquid infusion or decoction, add one and 1/2 pounds of sugar or 1 pound of honey, place in pan and heat until sugar or honey is melted, cool and store. Syrups will keep for 8 months to 1 year, or longer if refrigerated and sterile equipment is used, and alcohol or glycerine added as additional preservative.

Steam: Breathing in the vapors of an herbal infusion that is high in essential oils is a good way to treat respiratory problems. Inhalations can provide invaluable symptom relief, while other remedies taken internally are for more long-term treatment. To prepare an inhalation, make an infusion with the required herbs. Alternately, add 5-10 drops of essential oil into a small bowl of steaming hot water. Essential oils are the most convenient to use. Cover the head with a large heavy towel, and inhale the volatile oils for 5-15 minutes. Inhalations can be done 3 times a day or more.

Herbs for Children

There are many herbal treatments that are safe and effective for use with children of all ages. Here I will deal with the childhood illnesses and problems I am most often asked about.

The most important factor in dealing with any illness, whether acute or chronic, is diet. A proper diet goes a long way to alleviating problems and illnesses that stem from inadequate nutrition. Were you aware that medical studies are proving that diet can profoundly affect illness in children? It has also been proven that a lot of dietary factors are responsible for worsening such problems as Attention Deficit Disorder (ADD), hyperactivity, asthma, and others. A child who is getting what his or her body needs through good nutrition is going to develop more normally, be less prone to illness, and the duration of common illnesses is shortened.

Remember too that our children today are under a lot of stress, just as us adults are. Peer pressures, pressures in the classroom, dealing with separation anxieties and broken marriages are just some of the things creating stressful situations for our youngsters. This stress can manifest itself in many mysterious physical and mental ailments. Teaching your children when young how to meditate and relax is an important building block for their young lives, and is a useful tool that they will carry with them through adulthood.

Anxiety, Stress, Excitability

Externally, these problems can be alleviated with a warm herbal bath at bedtime. Combine a handful of lavender and a handful of chamomile in one quart of water. Bring to a boil, cover, and let steep for 15 to 20 minutes. Strain, then add the liquid to a warm bath for the child. This is good for colicky infants as well. Allow the child to bathe and relax in the warm water. Internally, a cup of the infusion of chamomile and/or scullcap can be very beneficial and calming.

Chickenpox
Chickenpox usually strikes in young children, but older ones do get it as well. To relieve the itching that usually makes the pox so unbearable, you can make a decoction of chickweed, comfrey, and rosemary. Apply the warm mixture with a clean cloth. Don't rub, as this will irritate the sores and can cause them to leave scars, but gently pat the solution on. Allow to air dry. This can be applied several times per day to relieve the itching. Internally, the child may benefit from a mild infusion of echinacea, catnip, chickweed, and yarrow. After the illness, and after any illness, the

child's digestive system will benefit from acidophilus, or a cup of yogurt, to aid getting the beneficial bacteria in the digestive system back in balance.

Colds

Most of the same herbs used to treat colds in adults can also treat colds in children. You will want to reduce the dosages, however, or make milder infusions than normal. Steam or inhalant therapy can also help, using essential oils of lavendar, tea tree, eucalyptus, and/or peppermint. Make sure the child is getting plenty of vitamin C in their daily diet for the duration of the cold.

Colic

Colic is torture for both the baby and the parent. There are easy ways to alleviate the problem, however. Give the baby a small amount of peppermint, chamomile, or catnip infusion in a bottle at the first sign of distress. It also helps to give the baby a warm bath that has lavender essential oil added. The vapors have a calming, soothing affect on baby and parent. Breastfeeding mothers will want to add some fennel to their diet for a couple of days to help alleviate the colic.

Cough

Coughs in children are common, and usually accompany many of the normal childhood illnesses. A cough that continues for several days, or increases in severity, should be immediately checked by a physician to rule out other diseases. A mild infusion of mullein and coltsfoot usually helps the mild cough. Horehound and/or ginger can be added if a stronger combination is needed for older children. The child can also benefit from chest rubs of tea tree oil or peppermint oil. Both should be diluted in olive or sesame oil, and remember to do a patch test first to determine sensitivity. Inhaling the vapors of the essential oil of lavender, and/or a warm bath that includes lavender oil, can also help clear a cough. Cut back or eliminate dairy products in children that have a lot of mucous with their coughs, as dairy often adds to the production of mucous.

Diaper Rash

This is a common problem that is easy to deal with. It is usually caused by irritating diapers, prolonged contact with wet or dirty diapers, or even a reaction to the soap used to wash cotton diapers. Some foods and juices ingested by the infant can raise acid levels in the urine and stool, causing a skin reaction. Wash the baby thoroughly and dry thoroughly at each diaper change.. Leaving the diaper off for a while each change can also help clear up the rash. You can also add to that mixture comfrey and/or chickweed.

Diarrhea

Diarrhea can cause dehydration rapidly in small infants and very young children. It can be treated with a mild infusion of meadowsweet, rosemary, and/or red raspberry.

If diarrhea continues for more than three days, or is accompanied by blood in the stool, or severe cramping, seek emergency medical care immediately.

Hyperactivity, ADD
There is strong evidence that chemicals such as heavy metal pollutants, dietary allergies such as to wheat, corn, dairy, etc., and artificial colorings, preservatives, or flavorings, play a role in these problems. As such, you will want to treat by supporting both the nervous system and the liver, aiding in detoxification. A treatment plan should consist of chamomile, gotu kola, scullcap, red clover, milk thistle, and gingko biloba. A daily supplement of flax seed and/or grape seed oil has also shown to be beneficial. The herbal bath above can help, as well as inhaling or massaging with a calming essential oil such as lavendar. And most important, look at changing the diet to one that supports the body. Natural diet is best. Eliminate foods that could cause an allergic reaction, and add them back to the diet one at a time, watching for any changes in the child's behavior. Be sure the child gets adequate amounts of zinc and B-complex vitamins as well.

Impetigo
Internally give a combination of echinacea, chickweed, and astragalus 3 to 4 times per day. Reduce the child's intake of dairy, red meats, and peanut butter, as all have been shown to irritate this illness. Wash the sores carefully with an infusion made of calendula several times per day.

Influenza
Flu can be treated internally with boneset, fenugreek, peppermint, echinacea, and mullein. Eucalyptus or tea tree oil can be inhaled to open blocked sinus passages, or rubbed on the chest to help open the bronchial tubes. Additional vitamin C and zinc are also beneficial.

Lice
Lice can be treated by placing drops of tea tree oil on a fine toothed comb, and comb the hair thoroughly every day for two weeks. Wash the hair nightly with a mild shampoo that has oil of thyme and tea tree oil added. Alternatively, you can mix together 4 cups of apple cider vinegar, 4 cups of water, 1/2 ounce oil of thyme; use nightly as a shampoo.

Measles
Measles is usually treated herbally in the same manner as chicken pox. Eye strain and discomfort is common with the measles, so keep the child in a darkened room. A mild infusion of eyebright may be used to ease discomfort in the eyes. This can be used as a wash for the older child, or for young children you can soak a clean cloth in the eyebright infusion and apply as an external compress over the eyes.

Mumps
Mumps can be treated internally with a combination of echinacea, clover, chamomile, and peppermint. Externally, fresh chopped ginger applied as a compress can alleviate the pain of the swelling. Gentle massage of the swollen areas with chamomile oil is also beneficial. Inhaling eucalyptus oil also helps.

Teething
Teething pain can be soothed by giving a chamomile and/or lemon balm infusion internally. Mix a teaspoon of powdered slippery elm bark with a little water to make a paste, and rub it gently on the gums.

Tonsillitis
Tonsillitis can be treated with echinacea, mullein, chamomile, and sage internally. A gargle of salt water, honey or agave and lemon (if the child is over the age of three), or sage infusion can greatly ease the discomfort.

Flower Essences

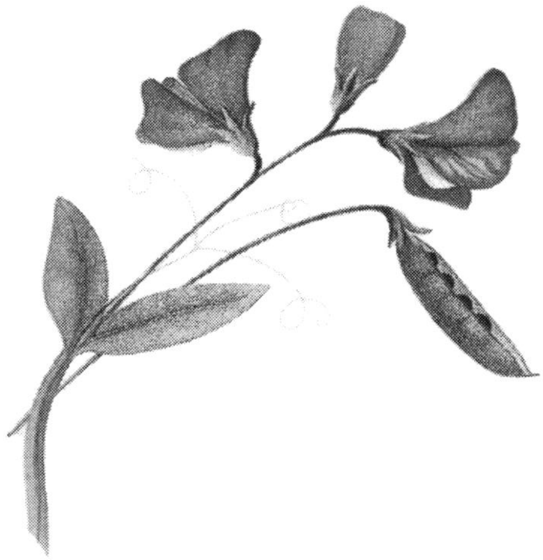

What are Flower Essences?

Flower Essences or Remedies are diluted extracts of various flowers which are preserved and usually taken by mouth by people and animals for various discomforts. Flower Remedies are a vibrational remedy. Therefore, flower remedies work alongside sound therapy, color therapy, aura healing and the like on the subtle energy fields of the body. However, this should not be understood to mean that there are no visible results. People who regularly use flower remedies and essences know their effectiveness and use flower remedies for numerous malaises. Results are seen with flower essences when taken over a period of time. However, one can begin to see the effects right away. Often people use affirmations along with each daily dose, and of course, simply the act of taking the essences reminds them of their desire to correct whatever difficulty they are experiencing.

This in itself may have some restorative powers. Most people who use flower essences feel that they experience big shifts in their lives, always in a very positive manner. Unfortunately, no scientific studies have been done at all on flower essences, so we cannot verify their effectiveness from a scientific point of view.

Then again, this is true for almost everything that is somewhat spiritual in nature. There simply is no scientific way to prove the spiritual (at least not quite yet).

Nevertheless, we cannot be sure that it is the actual flower or plant that is having an effect on our bodies (mental, physical or spiritual). All we know is that a difference is apparent. In a similar vein, doctors have shown us that placebos can be quite effective, and yet scientists dismiss them so easily. Should not we take the time to heal the whole person, mind body and soul? This is what flower essences strive to do. It should be understood that Flower Remedies and Flower Essences are for all practical purposes, one and the same. The difference in name comes from the association of the word 'flower remedy' to Dr. Edward Bach's life work. However, you may use the word interchangeable as most do. Many refer to Bach Flowers as "remedies" while most other groups maintain they create "essences", not remedies.

The Life and Work of Edward Bach

Dr. Bach grew up in Birmingham, England. From an early age, Back showed a keen interested in the human condition. Bach studied medicine in the University College Hospital, London. His biographers state that Bach spent much time by the bedside of his patients contrary to most of his colleagues. Thus he came to sense that the real cause of ill health was their worries and upsets, rather than pure physical ills. Bach was a homeopathic physician. He followed his intuition to understand the relationship between disease and people. Edward Bach believed as many holistic practitioners do today, that disease is the result of imbalances in the body at the soul level.

Dr. Bach's goal in life was to find a way to heal physical, mental and emotional imbalances. Edward Bach started his career as allopathic (orthodox) doctor. He began working in 1915 at University College Hospital in London specializing gin bacteriology. Only two years later he became ill and resigned from his position. After two years of illness, he recovered and then began working at the London Homeopathic Hospital. This is where his interest in holistic methods really accelerated.

Through the years, Dr. Bach worked with many patients in hospitals and in his own practice located on Harley Street. Bach was especially influenced by the vitalist tradition in healing. This philosophy holds that the functions of a living organism are derived from a vital principle beyond the mere physio-chemical forces with an emphasis on a stronger relationship to natural cures and herbal medicine.

Dr. Edward Bach was fascinated by nature and the outdoors. His deep love for nature combined with his goals of helping to heal, inspired him to find qualities in flowers and plants that resembled traits or qualities in human beings.
In his first year of working with flowers and patients, he found three plants that he

experimented with. He discovered Impatience, Mimulus and later Clematis growing in the countryside of England. He returned to London and tried these different plants with his patients. He found for example, that Impatience helped with irritability and tension. He found that the three flowers helped with different afflictions and this was the beginning of Dr. Bach's Remedies. In 1929, Bach started to pursue the effects of the extracts of the plants exclusively. He observed every detail of his patients and then searched for plants that matched his patients' needs.

His work was guided by intuition and his inner wisdom. He left London and moved to Cromer, Wales. Here he spent all his time with plants, studying every minute detail about them. He would sit with them, receive impressions and study them in depth. Although it may seem surprising to us, Dr. Bach was able to intuitively learn what effects a flower (or plant) could have by this method. This was the very beginning of what we call "Plant Signatures" or the "Doctrine of Signatures". A plant signature is a sort of 'clue' given by the plant in order for humans to be able to select that plant based on their needs. This could be color, odor, shape etc. All clues as to how the plant should be used. It was thought that God had left us a sign, so that we would be able to cure our maladies.

In spring and summer of every year, he searched for his remedies and prepared them. In winter he spent advising those people who came and sought out his help. What is interesting is that Dr. Bach claims that right before he found each remedy, he physically endured each of the malaises the remedies treat and was able to affect a cure based on the remedies he ingested.

By 1932, Bach had 12 of his remedies. The rest were found at Mt. Vernon in Oxfordshire. There, he completed his life work, and died at the relatively young age of 50. Dr. Bach originally created thirty eight remedies. Each essence works to treat a specific ailment.

Bach Remedies and other Essences

Bach Remedies are certainly the first if not the most popular remedies known today. The Dr. Edward Bach Centre in the UK composed this list of the 38 remedies discovered by Dr. Bach. These remedies are directed at a particular characteristic or emotional state. It's usually a good idea to start your study of Flower Essences with Bach Remedies as they are the most well-known and readily available. These remedies (as well as all others) can be used alone (which is often seen as the most effective as it's more focused on one particular imbalance) or in combination

Agrimony - mental torture behind a cheerful face. This remedy is used for people who tend to hide their true feelings. They may have fears and insecurities and yet, they never let others on to their suffering. They feel they may make others unhappy or concerned about them by sharing their true feelings. These people never complain and always put on a cheerful face. They are usually highly sensitive and take care in not disturbing others. Their biggest desire is for complete harmony in everything they do. It may seem difficult to get close to this person as they never want to show their true thoughts or feelings, always disguised under a smile and happy countenance.

Aspen - fear of unknown things, general anxiety (without a known cause) or apprehension; nervousness of seemingly ‘normal’ situations and things. Aspen is used in the case of a presenting fear with an unknown cause. Your 2 year old child for example may be terrified of vacuum cleaners, since s/he may not be able to tell you why or possibly does not even know why, you can use Aspen.

Beech – intolerance. Beech can be used in any situation where a person isn’t tolerant to another, a situation or another living thing. Beech was described by Dr. Bach as the remedy for people who 'feel the need to see more good and beauty in all that surrounds them”. It is for those who quickly pass judgment on others.

Centaury - the inability to say 'no' . Many people use Centaury with fascinating success. People can feel run down and walked on by others and yet they do not have the confidence or capability for whatever reason to say no. Centaury helps with that profoundly. People who give their all constantly and whom often play victim, willingly or unwillingly will greatly benefit from Centaury. These people are usually very giving souls who are easily used by others who have strong wills.

Cerato - lack of trust in one's own decisions. This is for the person who does not trust himself fully and constantly seeks the advice of others, thinking it will be better than the advice that comes from deep within. They may go back and forth a lot or generally lack faith in themselves. Cerato helps the person to trust their inner guidance and awareness.

Cherry Plum - for those with the fear of losing control of thoughts and actions and therefore doing negative things or things they do not ethically approve of. This can come about when a person feels pushed to the limit and highly stressed and is ready to explode; our emotions may feel dangerous and consuming or overwhelming. Cherry Plum helps one realize that every event is a lesson and we can walk through it gracefully.

Chestnut Bud - failure to learn from mistakes. Chestnut Bud teaches one to be a good learner and to learn from the past, and live in the present. This is a good remedy for bed wetting in children when all other factors are excluded. This can also be used for women who seem to get involved in the same types of unsatisfying relationships, whether personal or professional. An important thing to remember is that if we are not getting the desired results, then continuing to do the same things (even in a different guise) will not change anything.

Chicory - selfish, possessive love. Chicory is for anyone who feels a possessive need to be near and involved in a loved ones life to the detriment of the other. This could be the classic "mother hen" even if the 'child' is a grown adult.

Clematis - dreaming of the future without working in the present, lack of attention, unfocused. Clematis is for those who tend to live in a fantasy world, finding it more interesting than the present 'reality'. Clematis works as a bridge between the interior to the exterior worlds. This is an incredible essence for working with ADD/ADHD in children & adults alike. Clematis concentrates one's attention to the task at hand.

Crab Apple - the cleansing remedy, also for self-hatred. Crab Apple is used for those who feel that a perfect life, body, and thoughts are essential and without that, have feelings of uncleanliness or disgust with themselves.

Elm - overwhelmed by responsibility. Elm is wonderful for new parents, for an overworked person, for adolescences coming into young adulthood. There are a lot of changes going on and more responsibility at the same time. Usually a very temporary condition, any person feeling overwhelmed may benefit from the use of Elm.

Gentian - discouragement after a setback, even small insignificant details. This type of person is very grounded in and bound to the physical, they seek physical evidence for everything. If they have lack of evidence, they are easily discouraged.

Gorse - hopelessness and despair. Gorse is good for people who feel as though they cannot go on. Many, although certainly not all people who are chronically ill, are in a Gorse state.

Heather - self-centeredness and self-concern. This is an excellent remedy for those who constantly need to talk about themselves, or tell you their own story in life. These are really emotionally needy people and they seek attention. Heather is commonly a temporary condition. Sometimes when people go through a particular trying period, they have a strong need to talk about it to whomever will listen.

Holly – envy, jealousy and hatred. Holly is for those who feel lacking in love and therefore are envious towards others. The underlying issue is that these people do not really love themselves enough and this is projected onto others as other having more.

Honeysuckle - living in the past, stuck in a world of unrealized potentials or the memory of a lost loved one. Honeysuckle helps people to live fully in the present moment.

Hornbeam - procrastination, tiredness at the thought of doing something, general fatigue in even the thought of making it through the day. Hornbeam gives the enthusiasm and motivation.

Impatiens – impatience for others taking their time and impulses to act quickly. General behavior is rushed and this person rarely takes the time to slow down and enjoy life.

Larch - lack of confidence, low self esteem.

Mimulus - fear of known things. Person may be quite sensitive to general things that don't seem to bother others. Mimulus helps people remember that their fearfulness has become a habit and helps break the habit of being in a state of fear.

Mustard - deep gloom for no reason, sudden depression without a known cause. Sometimes we are overcome with feelings of depression and sadness in life and we may not know why. Mustard can break the dark heavy clouds and help us see the light once more.

Oak - the plodder who keeps going past the point of exhaustion. On the surface it may appear that these people are go-getters, who never stop. They take care of business that needs to be attended to and take care of all the details and responsibilities. Deep inside these people are exhausted and the use of the Oak remedy helps them slow down and realize that they too can enjoy life and share their burden.

Olive - mental or physical exhaustion, this could be after physical illness, lack of proper nutrition, having young children, working at a particularly demanding job, or intense personal work. Olive helps people listen to their bodies and their own needs: physical, emotional and mental.

Pine – guilt for mistakes and even others mistakes. For those who are never satisfied with themselves. Pine teaches self-acceptance.

Red Chestnut - over-concern for the welfare of loved ones. Red Chestnut is for those who worry constantly about loved ones and let their imaginations run wild with negative thoughts of what might happen. This remedy encourages positive thinking even in difficult situations.

Rock Rose - terror and fright. Rock Rose is for any circumstance which seems to change your world and for situations in which you feel frightened and unable to control any outcome whatsoever. Rock Rose helps you to positive action.

Rock Water - self-denial, rigidity and self-repression. Rock water is for those who are extremely hard on themselves. Rock Water teaches open-mindedness and flexibility.

Scleranthus - inability to choose between alternatives. For those with mood swings or who cannot make a decision, scleranthus teaches flexibility and balance.

Star of Bethlehem – past or present trauma or shock. Star of Bethlehem teaches us to integrate experiences into our present lives and learn from them.

Sweet Chestnut - Extreme mental anguish, when everything has been tried and there is no light left.

Vervain - over-enthusiasm with one's own belief system. Enthusiasm tends towards obsession.

Vine - dominance and inflexibility. .Vine is especially for those with a dictator type personality. It's very good with children who seem to dominate their parents with a controlling personality.

Walnut - protection from change and unwanted influences, Walnut is for those who are easily influenced by others (even well meaning friends) and therefore do not make all the positive changes they wish to make. Walnut is the second most popular essences in The USA. We have the potential to experience much change, and yet sometimes we are held back by well meaning family and/or friends who fear for us. Walnut can ease the stress we feel about leaving the old and starting with something new.

Water Violet – pride, independence and aloofness. Water Violet teaches those who are loners and reserved to share intimately with others without losing their own independence.

White Chestnut - unwanted thoughts and mental arguments which can cause loss of sleep. Constantly turning problem over in the mind without focusing on solutions. White Chestnut teaches balance.

Wild Oat - uncertainty over one's direction in life, for those who have no feel they lack purpose. Wild Oat teaches direction and focus in life.

Wild Rose - drifting, resignation, apathy in life. Good for those who have been emotionally abused or hurt and have coped by erecting barriers to their heart and emotions.

Willow - self-pity and resentment, not seeing the real cause of the problem. Willow is for those who blames others, or society, for their issues, problems, and obstacles.

There is also a **Rescue Remedy,** (the number one seller in the USA) which is a combination remedy made up of five different remedies. Rescue remedy is great to carry around with you in case of emergencies. This does not of course mean you do not tend to the emergency; it just gives you extra help with the emotions at hand.

Truly by looking at the above list and carefully reading about the remedies, we can easily become overwhelmed. The best way to learn more about each remedy and indeed become truly familiar with it is to meditate on each individual remedy, perhaps one per evening or even one per week. This is best done by using a photo of the plant and preferably a bottle of the remedy. Read as much as you can about the particular essence, and then take those thoughts to dreamtime with you every night for one week. By the end of that week, you will be completely familiar with the essence.

Although the Bach Remedies are marked with an expiration date, most if not all practitioners believe that flower essences never expire. We are working with subtle energy here, a vibrational remedy, not a product that will lose its potency. The remedy has nothing to do with potency, and more is not better. We will look at this later in the course when we discuss children and essences.

Other Sources of Flower Remedies

After Dr. Bach's creations, several other associations have been created to further the development of flower remedies. Among the more well-known, you will find California Flower Essences who create their remedies with the essence of flowers grown locally in the region of the Sierra Nevada foothills. Richard Katz founded the

FES (Flower Essence Society) in 1979 and in 1980 and Patricia Kaminski joined the organization as co-director. Today they estimate that 50,000 practitioners use flower essences in their healing work all over the world. FES has over 103 flower essences available at present. This not-for-profit organization is quite science oriented. Striving to make the use of flower essences more scientific and accepted as a more mainstream modality. They have done several studies themselves on depression and other related issues using flower essences. However, as stated before, no outside organized scientific body has undertaken any known scientific studies. The FES maintains a fourfold purpose to their organization:

1. To promote plant research and clinical research on the therapeutic effects of flower essences;

2. To train practitioners and spread knowledge of the use of flower essences throughout the world with seminars

3. To disseminate publications about flower essence therapy to practitioners and to the general public; and

4. To provide a communication and a referral network for those who are teaching, researching, or practicing in the field of flower essence therapy.

The society's Yarrow Environmental Solution pictured above, is effective in protecting against harmful environmental conditions such as pollution, radiation and other hazards. FES creates many wonderful essences which all merit close study and inspection. Please see the net links for a detailed list of their essences and studies.

Dosages

Dosages will vary but an average dosage is about 3-4 drops, 4 times a day, under the tongue directly or drank in a glass of water. It seems best to take the essences upon rising, twice throughout the day (but not with food) and once before retiring. It's a good idea to either state an affirmation while you take the essence or take some time and focus your intention on why you are taking the essence. I find it especially effective for children to state an affirmation, even if they are too little too understand the exact meaning, it remains within their consciousness as they grow and learn the meaning of the words. You may also use the essences in bath water or to spray in a room or spray on yourself.

It's the frequency of taking the dosages that creates the dedication to the process and the devotion necessary for the inner reflection and changes to take place. It's not advised to increase dosage amounts if one needs a higher dosage, but rather to increase dosage frequency. So if you feel you need more of the essence, take it 6 or even 8 times a day until you're feeling better. But do not increase your dosage amount (3-4 drops each dose). Because we are working with subtle energies, more will not make the difference, but increased frequency will. You can reduce the frequencies as you see the shifts and improvements in your life. If the condition requiring the essences is chronic, the flower essence should be used for at least one month.

If however the imbalance is temporary or acute, only a few doses may be enough to affect the desired shift. Children and older people seem especially sensitive to flower essences. Therefore by simply adjusting the dosages to between 1 and 3 times a day, the needed change will take place. At any point when you are taking the essences, when you feel as though the energetic shift has taken place, simply stop taking the essence. This goes for treating anyone in the family. When you or they feel they are better, you can recommend they stop taking the essence. Flower essences can be used with any other type of treatment modality. As a matter of fact, flower essences can enhance any other type of healing work. It is used frequently by practitioners of bodywork and other types of healing such as Reiki and Crystal healing.

The Doctrine of Signatures

A physician named Paracelsus originated the Doctrine of Signatures. It undoubtedly existed a long time even before that, but from written history we assume that the doctrine originated with him. He adopted the Latin phrase "similia simiibus curantur" meaning "like cures like". He believed that the "essence of the plant is similar to the essence of the disease, organ or constitution to which it is suited as medicine". The doctrine of signatures is simply about matching the similarities of a plant construct to a person's needs based on the plants qualities and traits. The doctrine of signatures holds that the personality and characteristics of a plant (including all parts of the plant, plus the color, odor and texture) are a statement about its medicinal qualities and properties. For example, an onion may induce watery eyes and sneezing when its odors are inhaled.

Therefore it is presumed to be beneficial for head colds with those symptoms. When you are in the presence of a flower or plant, look at it carefully. Spend time observing the petals, the stigma, the style, the nectary, the anthers and the stalk of the flower and also the way you feel in relation to the flower. Appreciate this beauty nature has created. Just as our bodies are to be considered temples for their magnificence, you will also easily see the wonder and magnificence of the flower and plant.

Helping Yourself and Others

By now, you completely understand the process of creating your own essences and hopefully you have taken the time to do at least one plant journey. As you continue to work with flower essences, you will highly develop your intuition. You will want to start by working with essences on yourself for quite a while before moving on to helping others outside your own family.

Choosing an essence for yourself can be done by several different methods. It can be an essence or flower you're particularly attracted too or that you feel some sort of connection with, you can use the Bach repertoire listed in the net links sections or you can refer back to the previous lessons where you learned about different flower essences and their properties. Finally, two especially effective ways to test which essences would be best are the pendulum and muscle testing. When using a pendulum, simply place the pendulum between your choices and ask the pendulum. If more than one essence is needed then you will have to continually test until you are able to get the right number of essences and which essences. You can also test for dosage quantities if you are unsure.

It's preferable to fill out a complete Flower Essence questionnaire and evaluate what's most seriously bothering you. Look at where you need help exactly in your life. What are the blocks? You may have several you're dealing with at the same time. You can choose to take several remedies (up to 5). However, it's a personal choice and some practitioners believe (as stated earlier) that taking so many makes one lose focus, and therefore motivation for self healing is diluted.

When sharing your knowledge with others, you should professionally refer to it as an 'assessment'. At no times are you to make claims that flower essences can 'cure' anything. If you do, you are likely to be charged for practicing medicine without a license. Holistic practitioners are not allowed to diagnose anything at all. To play it safe, refer the client to the claims that the manufacturers make or what can be found in a reference book. A good way to do this would be". When I was working on my certification, we discussed that (fill in the blank) may be helpful to your situation. I know its something that has helped me." In this way, you are not even coming close to doing anything that is reserved for health professionals.

There are many ways to learn about flower essences and become a 'practitioner'. Practitioner training is not regulated by any governing body. Flower essences as a career can be very rewarding. It's a profession where you are guaranteed to have continual learning and growth. It's quite spiritual in nature as you are aware and this in itself aids in your personal spiritual growth and evolution. As a practitioner you must abide by ethics as any healer would.

You can also explain to the individual that flower essences are a bit like herbal medicines in that they contain certain diluted elements of the flowers that aid in healing. Share your success stories and your personal experiences with the remedies.

For users of flower essences and for practitioners, it's important to know (and explain) about what is termed 'the healing crisis'. This is a short period of time, just after the start of taking a flower essence (or doing any other subtle energy work for that matter) that a person experiences a 'letting go' of suppressed emotions and feelings accompanied by a major shift in thought patterns. It's important to feel encouraged then when one experiences a healing crisis. This short lived situation terminates quickly and you have just witnessed the power in flower essences. It's a very positive move in the right direction.

Many emotional and mental traumas come in layers. That means you may have to use more than one cycle of remedy for a particular complaint. It may subside for a while, and then perhaps a small part will reappear. However, this is true with any type of healing work. All of us are like onions, we have many deep layers and there is no magical cure. We all have to work through our own issues.

Flower Essence Questionnaire

What is the current condition(s) or issues at present that have brought you to this consultation? How can I help?

Approximately when did these conditions begin?

Do you have any fears at present?

Describe your sleeping pattern:

Do you need constant outside approval?

Do you feel unrecognized by your who you are?

How do you deal with daily challenges?

Any addictions, dependencies, etc?

Describe yourself. How would others describe you?

Describe your personal concerns?

Anything significant that stands out from your childhood?

Using Flower Remedies with Animals

Today there is an incredible interest in using flower essences with animals. Some veterinarians use alternative therapies like Reiki and flower essences on pets and livestock with excellent results. Bach remedies are used by people worldwide and yet Bach himself insisted that his remedies could also be used effectively in treating plants and animals.

Bach remedies were already being used on animals as early as 1939. Nora Weeks, a colleague of Bach and who administrated the Centre upon Bach's death in 1936 and personally prepared the flower essences, stated "Animals suffer from moods in the same way as human beings, and so indicate their state of health. The Remedies help man and beast alike." Because Bach Remedies have been used for treatment on animals for the last 66 years, we will focus on Bach Remedies for animals in this section, although others are widely available. Flower essences are ideal as they are easy to administer and there are no harmful side effects. In addition, animals respond quite well and very quickly to flower essences.

It's important to know that our house pets often reflect our own personal moods and take on our own malaises. If we are undergoing a lot of stress for example, our beloved doggie or kitty may suddenly get a nasty ear infection. In effect, the animal takes on our stress and his or her own immune system defenses are lowered. Animals can express behaviors that communicate happiness or sadness and a whole other spectrum of emotions just as we do. These emotions are especially apparent when there is an imbalance. Sometimes a pet will express unhappiness at the owner's leaving and soil all over the house, a pet may be overly clingy or possessive. There may be separation anxiety, aggression or a number of other difficulties. An animal may experience trauma if it's taken from its mother too early or if it's abandoned in a kennel.

Bach Flower Remedies for Animals

Following are a list of Bach remedies that have been used successfully with animals. Experiment and see if they provide comfort and assistance to your pet friends. They are easiest administered by adding drops to their drinking water, but you can also place on their paws or mix them in with their food.

The recommended dosage is 4-6 drops up to three times a day. I have had much success with essences with my cats, and personally believe that it is the reason my cat, Hematite, survived a parasitic brain infection when the vet had no cure. I used crab apple in addition to an herbal tincture I made.

Agrimony:
Restores inner peace and contentment. This remedy is especially useful for pets who constantly try to please their owners, for anxious animals and anxiety that results in psychosomatic conditions (digestive problems, skin problems).

Aspen:
Remedies fears of an unknown cause. These fears may cause physical symptoms such as trembling with fear or urination.

Beech:
For intolerance. This is ideal for pets that need to be more flexible, for animals that do not like change, are easily annoyed or irritated.

Centaury: ideal for pets who need to be more assertive. For animals that work constantly at pleasing and show submissive behavior (urinating when petted etc).

Cherry Plum: good for aggressive behaviors such as biting and general violence towards humans or other animals.

Ceranto: ideal for animals that need to improve their self confidence, those who cannot act on their own initiative, have immature or inadequate social skills.

Cherry Plum: for uncontrollability, unwanted and/or compulsive behavior

Chestnut Bud: excellent for breaking bad habits, accident prone pets, constant sickness or any kind of repetition due to lack of learning from experience.

Chicory: for very possessive pets, constant attention seekers, jealous of others (animals or people).

Clematis: ideal for animals that are absentminded, spacey, do not concentrate or who are bored or disinterested.

Crab Apple: for cleansing the physical body and riding it of toxins, infections and feelings of uncleanliness. This remedy works on the physical body and has been used successfully in treatment of mange on dogs, cats and foxes.

Elm: helps feelings of inadequacy, overwhelmed by situations or training, difficulty adjusting to new demands.

Gentian: good for animals that are easily discouraged and give up right away. This would be a good remedy to use in training your animal is they give up easily. Helps with appetite and weakness after surgery.

Gorse: remedies hopelessness. Good for mothers who lose their offspring and other animals who feel great despair.

Heather: helps barking, noisy attention getting behavior, animals that suffer from separation anxiety and thus whine or cry a lot.

Holly: great for animals who lack trust, are jealous and tend to be aggressive due to this. Aggression can be directed either at another animal or a person.

Honeysuckle: Excellent for homesick animals or those who need to adjust to new situations, for those taken on vacation and cannot deal with the changes.

Hornbeam: a great remedy for restoring vitality and spunk! Helpful for animals suffering for terminal illnesses or animals who need help to revive activity after a prolonged period of sickness or confinement.

Impatiens: for animals that are irritable, impatient who need to be calmed and cooperative. This remedy is great for hyperactivity or animals that are constantly on edge. Also good for skin conditions and muscular pain. Good for dogs who take their owner for a walk instead of the other way around (constantly pulling on the leach)

Larch: for animals that lack confidence, are hesitant, who need coaxing to do something. For animals that are timid and shy.

Mimulus: for animals that are afraid of things (that are known) storms, dark, water, traffic, stairs, fireworks, being clipped, loud noises, visiting the vet, a bath, etc.

Mustard: For depression in animals without known cause. For animals who feel 'down'. When a pet suddenly shows signs of depression but owner doesn't know what's wrong, mustard is excellent.

Oak: Works to restore strength and resilience. Good for animals that are exhausted or working too hard. Oak is excellent for animals that show obsession behaviors or concealed weakness.

Olive: Ideal for fatigue due to exhaustion from an illness or some sort of strain. Helps regenerate, restore and makes them feel healthy again.

Pine: Ideal for guilt and helps restore a positive healthy attitude.

Red Chestnut: Good for animals who are overprotective and fear for others (their offspring for example). This remedy can be used for animals who are overprotective with their owners as well, for mother animals who won't allow anyone close to their offspring.

Rock Rose: For animals who are high strung and often show sheer terror or panic. Rock Rose helps to restore calmness and helps with courage.

Rock Water: Good for animals that feel repressed, are inflexible and insistent. These animals may need help to loosen up and adapt to new situations. Especially good for stubbornness and arthritic conditions.

Scleranthus: Ideal for hormone imbalances, animals with seizures or suffering from unknown illnesses, for travel sickness and inner ear problems. Scleranthus restores balance.

Star of Bethlehem: Helps all forms of shock and trauma: physical, mental and emotional. Trauma can be from long ago past or recent.

Sweet Chestnut: Great for animals who are have been mistreated, who suffer from mental anguish, mother animals that have experienced a difficulty birthing offspring. Good for suffering associated with various difficulties, illness, being in forced captivity, any situation that causes great stress and strain on the animal. Additionally sweet chestnut is helpful for animals who chew at their skin and fur, who have skin irritations due to mental conditions. This remedy is also helpful for wild animals placed in captivity for any reason.

Vervain: ideal for hyperactivity, impulsiveness and high strung animals. Great for pets with excessive energy.

Vine: Excellent for dominating animals who feel they are the boss! These pets are bullies to others, do not like discipline and are very territorial.

Walnut: Ideal for animals that have difficulty adapting to new situations or change. Walnut is highly effective after neutering, during weaning, changing houses, adjusting to new animals in the family or any other major life changes.

Water Violet: For animals who are reserved, introverted and detached. This remedy helps the animal become friendlier and open to others.

White Chestnut: This remedy is great for restlessness and inability to relax and sleep. Excellent for animals who constantly move their young and who have obsessive behavior.

Wild Oak: Good for lack of direction, helps channel energy and potentials. Wild oak is excellent for animals that do not seem to be living up to their abilities and helps animals settle down.

Wild Rose: For animals who have given up on life and the will to live and appear to derive no joy from living. This may be due to being abandoned, having a long standing illness.

Willow: Helps with resentment, sulkiness, and bad tempers. Good for cats who urinate around the house as a means of acting out, or animals that are not happy due to the arrival of a new family member (animal or human).

Rescue Remedy: This remedy is a combination of remedies and helps with any type of trauma or stress. This is good to have on hand at all times. I used this a lot when I first rescued my oldest female cat, Miss Piggy, from an abusive home condition.

Color & Light Therapy

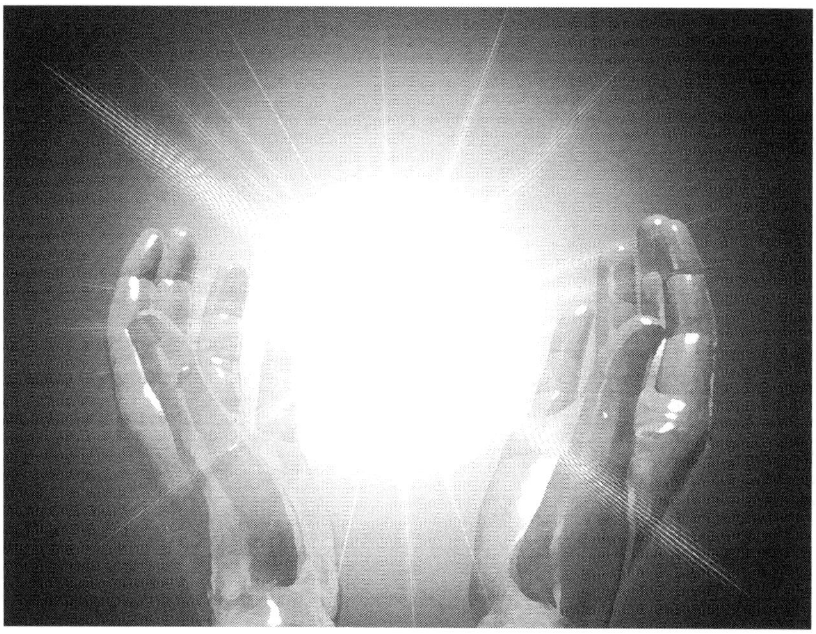

What is Color Therapy?

Colors are visible light energies of certain wavelengths. Photoreceptors in the retina, called cones, translate this energy into colors. When the energy of color enters our bodies, it stimulates the pituitary and pineal glands. This in turn affects the production of certain hormones, which in turn affect a variety of physiological processes. This explains why color has been found to have such a direct influence on our thoughts, moods, and behavior-an influence that many experts believe is distinctly separate from psychological and cultural factors. Color seems to have an effect even on blind people, who are thought to sense color as a result of energy vibrations created within the body.

Specific colors can also have an effect on specific diseases. These treatments have been shown to alter neurochemical production in the brain and this may account for their positive effects. Scientists now believe that the brain has specific responses to different frequencies of flashing light and the different frequencies of various colors. They point out that sleep problems can often be cured in one day by this method. Mood alteration takes a little longer - about one to two weeks of treatments.

Color therapy, also known as chromotherapy, is based on the premise that certain colors are infused with healing energies. The therapy uses the seven colors of the rainbow to promote balance and healing in the mind and body.

Origins

Color therapy is rooted in Ayurveda, an ancient form of medicine practiced in India for thousands of years. Ayurveda is based on the idea that every individual contains the five basic elements of the universe: earth, water, air, fire, and ether (space). These elements are present in specific proportions unique to an individual's personality and constitution. When these elements are thrown out of balance through unhealthy living habits or outside forces, illness results. Ayurvedic medicine uses the energies inherent in the colors of the spectrum to restore this balance. We will cover more about Ayurveda in a later chapter.

Color therapy was also used in ancient Egypt and China. In traditional Chinese medicine (TCM), each organ is associated with a color. In qigong, healing sounds are also associated with a color, which in turn corresponds to a specific organ and emotion.

The Meaning of Colors

All matter emits vibrations. A human being also radiates subtle emanations of everything of which he is composed. A person with extra sensitive sight is able to see the colors of this ray at a certain angle and speaks of them as the person's aura.

RED has the lowest vibration, being therefore the coarsest and most physically vitalizing: its place is just above the heat vibrations, and it is heat-giving in itself. Astrologers tell us that the "planetary color" of Mars is red and has dynamic power over iron. It is iron that is responsible for our red blood-without it we would have some sort of pale liquid in our veins. Red is the color associated with the root chakra. It is the lowest of the seven colors, and it belongs to the lowest of the seven notes of the musical scale, which is C: and most martial music is in the key of C.

ORANGE is the second color in the spectrum. This beautiful color is associated with the Sun, and has also a warming and invigorating effect. But whereas red is stimulating to the body and the blood, orange is stimulating to the emotions. Orange is the color associated with the sacral chakra. Its musical note is D. Melodies in that key often have emotional appeal. The metal associated with the Sun is Gold.

YELLOW is the third color of the spectrum. Yellow is the color associated with the solar plexus chakra. Wisdom is said to be conferred by Mercury and its color yellow. Buddha always dressed his priest in Yellow. This color has stood for wisdom and intellect throughout the ages. Yellow lamps or glass windows stimulate the nerves of the brain and the body. They should not be used by highly nervous subjects. Yellow is third color in the spectrum. It corresponds to the musical note of E. When seen in the human aura yellow if dark and crude, tells of deceit and cowardice, but if pale and luminous it shows high wisdom and intellectuality.

GREEN is the fourth color which stands in the center of the scale of seven colors. It is the color associated with the heart chakra. Green gives stability, endurance and quietude. Its action is to cool the blood and animate the nerves. Green belongs to fourth note of the musical scale, F.

BLUE Pale blue in the aura represents devotion, while dark blue shows fanaticism. Blue is the color that corresponds to the throat chakra. The musical note of blue is G.

INDIGO is the sixth color of the scale. It is the color associated with the brow or third eye chakra. In the aura it shows dignity and high aspirations.
The musical note is A.

VIOLET is the seventh and last color of the spectrum. It represents the seventh and highest quality a person attains- noble spiritual aspiration. Violet is the color associated with the crown chakra. Its musical note is B. It cools the nerves, is magnetic and antiseptic.

PINK has a soothing effect on the body, relaxing muscles. Because it has been found to have a tranquilizing effect on aggressive and violent people, pink is often used in prisons, mental wards/institutions, hospitals, and juvenile and drug centers.

BROWN is the color of the earth and holds us to the earth and materialistic thoughts.

GRAY is neutral and useful as a background to other colors.

WHITE/LIGHT absorbs all the rays and is therefore cooling and restful.

BLACK absorbs them all and is warm, although neutralized.

When working with color therapy (chromotherapy) keep in mind the color associations that are associated with the energy (chakra) points of the body as well as the systems or organs that are associated with that specific color. There are many levels of healing, not just the physical level. Colors and energy healings work on the mental, emotional and spiritual levels as well.

Using "Solarized" Water

This is a simple and cheap way of applying color to the body. Water, when exposed to sunlight in a colored container for at least an hour become irradiated and takes on some of the vibrational energy of that particular color. Safe food colorings can also be used, or you can wrap a clear container with a cellophane, paper, or cloth of the color you need. This is called solarized water. Simply drink (solarized water should always be sipped) this water at regular intervals throughout the day. Refrigerate after making. If you wish to make color elixirs for clients to take with them, you can also add a high proof alcohol, such as vodka, to the water mixture. Typically, you use 25% alcohol to 75% water. This will preserve the elixir for several months.

COLORS AND THE CONDITIONS THEY TREAT

Abdominal Cramps	Yellow, Lemon
Aches (ear)	Turquoise
Aches (head)	Blue, Green
Aches (muscles)	Pastel Orange
Acne	Pink, Red-violet
AIDS	Red, Indigo, and violet
Alzheimer's	Royal Blue, Blue-Purple, and Yellow
Anemia	Red
Anorexia	Blue
Arthritis	Red, Violet, Blue-Violet
Blood Ailments	Red
Blood Pressure (high)	Blue, Green
Blood Pressure (low)	Red, Red-Orange
Burns	Green
Cancer	Alternate use of Indigo and Green
Colds	Red
Cramps	Green
Depression	Yellow
Diabetes	Indigo
Epilepsy	Green
Fevers	Green
Gall bladder	Orange
Gout	Violet
Hay fever	Violet
Headaches	Green
Heart conditions	Red
Hyperactivity	Purple
Indigestion	Yellow
Insomnia	Blue
Kidneys	Violet
Liver	Green
Menopause	Green
Nausea	Blue
Nervousness	Blue
Obesity	Red
Ovaries	Blue
Sinusitis	Green and Blue
Sore throat	Green
Ulcers	Green and Purple

Preparing for a Session

If you are already skilled in Reiki or any other holistic art, feel free to do whatever preparations you are comfortable with before the session. Balancing can be done with the client standing, sitting, or laying down, so decide what will be of most comfort for them.

I highly recommend that you purify your working space with incense, oils, and/or meditation/prayer. Feel free to invite your guides/angels/God to assist you with this work. If nothing else, make sure that you visualize a protective white light around you and your client for the work ahead. Either silently or aloud declare that your intent in balancing the chakras is for the highest good for all parties involved.

Ask your client to decide what position they are going to be most comfortable in. They need not remove any clothing! It may be advised that they remove their shoes or jewelry, but absolutely no nudity is required or necessary for the balancing.

If you will be treating someone distantly, it may help if you have a photo or can visualize what they look like- otherwise meditation on their name, address, and what you do know about them will be important for the procedure to take affect.

Please view your manual to become familiar with the chakras, their properties, locations, etc. When you are confident that you are familiar with this material, it will then be time for you to begin to treat yourself or others. Gather your stones and mists. You need not use these items, but their colors and properties are especially helpful for beginners. There are special incenses, oils, and other chakra products available to assist you. You may contact me for more info on how to obtain these optional items.

Sound/Music Therapy

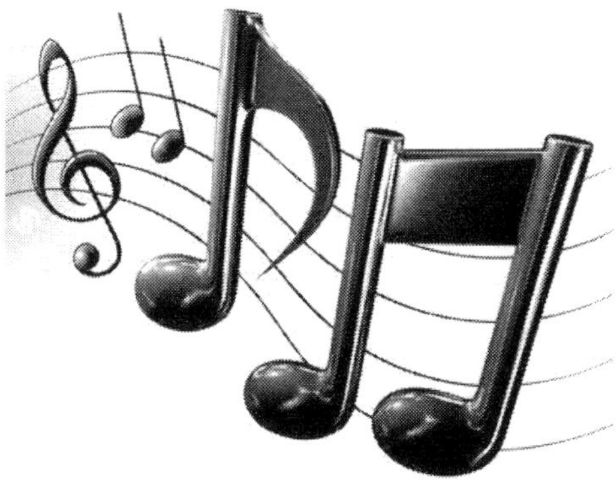

What is Sound Therapy?

Sound/Music Therapy is the use of music and music-related strategies, by a qualified music therapist, to assist or motivate a person towards specific, non-musical goals. Music therapists use their training as musicians, clinicians, and researchers to effect changes in cognitive, physical, communication, social, and emotional skills. Music therapists work in a variety of settings, including educational, medical, psychiatric, wellness, and holistic health facilities.

Sound Therapy is the prescribed use of music and musical interventions in order to restore, maintain, and improve emotional, physical, physiological, and spiritual health and well being. Within this definition are the key elements, which define interventions as music therapy.

Sound or Music Therapy is the primary therapeutic tool. Using music to establish a solid relationship, the music therapist then works to improve the client's physical and mental functioning through carefully structured activities. Examples can include singing, listening, playing instruments, composition, moving to music, and music and imagery exercises.

A music therapist's education and training combines studies of the music's effect on behavior, the client's strengths and weaknesses, and the therapeutic goals. And its effect on the body, mind and soul.

Music therapy is received by a client and it targets a wide range of populations and ages. It works towards specific therapeutic goals and objectives. Goal area includes communicative, academic, motor, emotional, and social skills. It is important to be aware that while clients may develop their musical skills during treatment, these skills are not the primary concern of the therapist. Rather it is the affect such musical development might have on the client's physical, psychological and socio-economical functioning.

What Types of People do Music Therapists Work With?

You can find music therapists working with a wide variety of people. Some examples include the mentally ill, the physically handicapped, those who have been abused, the elderly including those suffering from Alzheimer's and dementia, the terminally ill, the mentally retarded and the developmentally delayed, the traumatically brain injured, those with learning disabilities, as well as those persons who do not suffer from a clinical diagnosis.

How Sound Therapy Works

Our body has an "energetic system" as well as a "physical system". The "energetic system" has also been called variously chi, subtle energy, vital energy, and prana. Energies are primordial. They are the basic foundation of all existence. Although this idea is new to Westerners, Oriental medicine has shown for thousands of years that when the body's vortices of energy are in perfect balance, the result is a stronger vital force resulting in superior physical, mental, emotional and spiritual health. When our energies are blocked, heavy, veiled, weak, out-of-balance, dulled or altered, we may find potential conditions of disease.

Forms of sound, color, light, toning and music have the capacity to "tune-up" and balance the energy system, making it more efficient. Pain is eased, stress reduced and depression lifted. Personalities liven up and become more vibrant. The mind becomes clearer, resulting in increased creativity and ability to make major decisions. The emotions become more stable. The spirit is more peaceful. Greater joy and better health are found in the process.

The process is not magical but rather quite common in music therapies. A close analogy can be found in some forms of ultrasonic stimulation particularly in cases where some tissues remain neutral and others are stimulated. "Intuitives" report that many dull colors (our "wounds" or causal forces) are released from the energy field as we listen to the tones of MMST. Other colors remain unchanged.

The word Hue (when referring to a color) or Hu (when referring to sound) carries with it a tremendously high vibration capable of breaking up patterns that inhibit wholeness or health on any level. When we take full responsibility for our lives we will recognize that we are the ones responsible for creating or accepting the patterns that either help or hinder us.

Our focus activates these patterns and over a period of time we create grooves in our minds somewhat like a record or a CD. The patterns that we create start on the Mental level and usually are accepted unconsciously as an attitude. As children we are very good at doing this. Once we have experienced 'enough' of a pattern or patterns and are ready to change them we can invite the higher vibration of Hue (Hu) into our lives. Each color hue has a matching sound vibration. Each color hue has a word that exactly matches its quality or essence and this 'word' can also be said to be an attitude that we adopt. It's like a musical massage, the result is deep relaxation fast. The full body surround sound system is state of the art and the inner journey is out of this world.

Like the union and merging of Yoga, Sound Therapy incorporates the use of music, breath and meditation to relax and heal the mind and body allowing your spirit to flow freely. This brings about an awesome feeling of well-being and happiness to say nothing of the stress management.

How Long Has Music Therapy Been Used?

The Monks were the first to discover Sound Therapy. But while music has been used as a therapeutic mean for centuries, music therapy did not emerge as an organized profession until 1950 with the establishment of the National Association for Music Therapy and the American Association for Music Therapy in 1971. When the two associations merged in 1998, the new acronym became AMTA. The American Music Therapy Association.

Qualifications

Music Therapists should have a basic background of music theory. They follow their practice with at least six months of training. Music therapists should also be board-certified by a Holistic Health Practitioner society like Healers Unite, WMA, or ACHH to name a few.

Where do Sound Therapists Work?

Sound therapists work in hospitals, nursing facilities, schools, treatment centers, hospices, and group homes, as well as in private practice. Music Therapy can be combined with other modalities of energy, frequency therapies such as Reiki, Reflexology or a Crystal Healing session.

What is the Bonny Method of Guided Imagery and Music?

This technique (known as GIM) was developed by music therapist Dr. Helen Bonny. It is a music-centered therapeutic process to access the human psyche and lead to self-actualization and healing. GIM involves imaging to music in an alternate state of consciousness while sharing the imagery experience with a trained guide/therapist. When used as a therapeutic tool, GIM can lead to a deep uncovering of hidden emotional responses and stimulate creative insights.

Improvisational Music Therapy

The improvisational model often includes Nordoff-Robbins, Clinical Orff Schulwerk, or other types of improvisational styles. The basic philosophy of the improvisational music therapy is that these techniques elicit client's responses from every level. It develops contact with the client within the context of the musical experience. The role of a music therapist in this model often works supportively, creating a musical emotional environment that accepts and enhances the client's responses. This method provides experiences for socialization, communication, and expression of feelings and emotions among group participants. The most common instruments used for this method are rhythm instruments and Orff instruments. The music therapist can also integrate movement, speech, and drama in this model.

Guided Imagery and Music

GIM is a technique in which the act of listening to classical music is combined with a relaxed state of mind and body in order to evoke imagery for the purpose of self-actualization. The imagery evoked reflects aspects of the self and is used by the client, with the aid of the therapist. GIM does not intend to cure or treat symptoms; rather it is in search of client's inner awareness. There is a belief that everyone can understand his or her problems and has the ability to overcome the problem within the self. Thus, GIM is based on humanistic therapy, influenced by Abraham Malsow and Jung.

Music Therapy facilitates the creative process of moving toward wholeness in the physical, emotional, mental, and spiritual self in areas such as: independence, freedom to change, adaptability, balance and integration. The implementation of Music Therapy involves interactions of the therapist, client and music. These interactions initiate and sustain musical and non-musical change processes which may or may not be observable. As the musical elements of rhythm, melody and harmony are elaborated across time, the therapist and client can develop relationships which optimize the quality of life. We believe Music Therapy makes a unique contribution to wellness, because human's responsiveness to music is unique.

Definition of Music Therapy

The following 'Joint Declaration of the 1982 International Symposium of Music Therapists' best describes "Music Therapy facilitates the creative process of moving toward wholeness in the physical, emotional, mental, and spiritual self in areas such as: independence, freedom to change, adaptability, balance and integration. The implementation of Music Therapy involves interactions of the therapist, client and music. These interactions initiate and sustain musical and non-musical change processes, which may or may not be observable. As the musical elements of rhythm, melody and harmony are elaborated across time, the therapist and client can develop relationships which optimize the quality of life. Music Therapy makes a unique contribution to wellness, because man's responsiveness to music so unique.

Tips for Using Sound in Therapy & Education

Use Silence. Once we know a piece of music, we notice when it is interrupted. You can use unexpected pauses in music to get the attention of students whose attention has wandered. Once you have their attention back, you can resume exactly where you left off -- like the pause button on a tape player. No verbal cues necessary, just silence.

Make Sure the Lyrics Fit the Music. When you are using songs to teach academic concepts -- especially to students with language delays -- be sure that the words and phrases in the song are pronounced, as they would be in speech. Often, when songs are combines with new words with a familiar melody the words get distorted. Many children with special needs learn speech through singing; if they learn to pronounce words incorrectly, it may take a long time to unlearn.

Use Quality Instruments. Rather than buying a "bargain" box filled with instruments that have a bad sound quality as well as being breakable. Choose a few high-quality instruments that your students can share. Try a paddle drum, rattles and a rainstick to start. All are visually interesting, appropriate for older as well as younger students, and have unique, intriguing sounds.

Use Music with Discretion. Do you hear your refrigerator buzzing? Most of us don't because we've gotten so used to it, we block it out. If music is an effective tool, use it when you most need it. Playing music all day won't make children smarter; it will just teach them to tune it out.

Include by Adapting. A few simple adaptations will help in including children with special needs in regular education music settings. If the class is learning to play the recorder, for example, the music teacher can identify one or two "pedal" tones for each piece: the child with special needs can play just those two notes on a recorder, or on a resonator bell, for example. Children who cannot participate in singing can play rhythm instruments to accompany their peers.

Use Live Music, You Can Sing! Live music is, in most cases, much more effective than recorded music. If you sing the songs, you can change the tempo and volume according to the mood and behavior of the class you can pause to allow time for responses or to cue attention (see above), and you can change the words to fit your lesson. You can sing. If you have trouble, (1) learn to sing in the range of your speaking voice – you'll hit more notes; (2) practice to the radio/tape/CD in your car – and if you're trying to learn a particular song, have a musical friend tape it for you so you can practice singing along; (3) sing louder and slower – you may not think you have a good voice, but your students will be far more responsive if you sing with conviction and enjoyment than quietly and quickly.

Benefits of Sound/ Music in a Healing Session

To serve as an audioanalgesic or sedative, or to otherwise positively affect biomedical or psychosocial states.

Example: a patient with chronic pain is taught to use music to (a) decreases the physiological results of stress, (b) distract attention from pain, and /or (c) alter the perception of time towards a decreased perception of pain. OR pediatric patients participate in a music therapy group, which boosts their immune systems' effectiveness.

To serve as the focus of attention and/or to structure exercise
Example: a woman uses music in labor and delivery that has been programmed according to her preferences and choice of birthing technique OR a patient uses music as a structure and motivation for physical therapy exercises

To initiate and enhance therapist/patient/family relationships
Example: a therapist develops a trust relationship with an adolescent by sharing in his favorite music OR a teenage (or otherwise "at-risk") mother is taught to nurture her child (before and after birth) through music.

To reinforce learning.
Example: a child is taught a self-care routine by a therapist who has embedded the steps in a song OR a group of patient composes a song together that which reinforces the principles of health that they are learning.

To provide auditory stimulation/feedback or mask ambient noise.
Example: a patient learns to control muscle tension (or other physiological stress indicators) through biofeedback – using music as the auditory cue OR music played in an intensive care nursery unit masks mechanical and electronic sounds.

To structure pleasurable and positive interpersonal interactions.
Example: the members of patient/family support groups utilize lyric discussion, songwriting, singing and instrumental improvisation to increase their trust and cooperation with each other and with the facilitator.

To serve as a reinforced structure for healthful changes in or lifestyle skills.
Example: a patient learns to play the piano – as an outlet for expression, and as an active alternative to more passive activities OR persons participating in exercise groups find them easier if music that is synchronized to their movements is used in the background.

To promote stress reduction/mind-body health in the medical staff.
Example: the staff on an Alzheimer's unit attend services to learn to use music for stress reduction – and stress reduction sessions are offered by the music therapist 15 minutes before each shift.

How to Conduct a Session

Music therapists draw from an extensive array of music activities and interventions. For example, the therapist and client might compose songs for the purpose of expression of feelings; one client might learn to play the piano for the purpose of improving fine motor skills, while another client might use instruments to improvise unspoken emotions. Music therapists may also use music and movement activities, singing, lyric discussion or music and imagery (including the Bonny Method of Guided Imagery and Music) to help.

Using Tuning Forks

The sounds of the tuning forks help balance the chakras in two ways. At the same time that the disharmonious conditions are being adjusted or removed, a sacred space is created for strengthening of the person's Higher Self connection or "Divine Blueprint". When an unbalanced energetic condition is removed, it is always wise to fill the void created with the highest aspect of Source that the person is willing to embrace. The sound waves from tuning forks, voice, recorded music, or crystal bowls emit a pure holographic template of radiant sound that builds a deeper connection with the Divine.

The pure tones of tuning forks produce a vibrational sound field that resonates the light body energy centers (chakras) and corresponding physical areas.

Another sound therapy tool is the singing bowl. Much like tuning forks, these bowls are created in varying shapes and sizes to allow for a specific musical tone to be made. They can also be used for meditation and concentration.

Both tuning forks and singing bowls are wonderful additions to your practice, but can be rather expensive and are not required for successful sound healing. I suggest, especially for the new practitioner, to stick with music, small hand tools such as drums, and your own voice.

Using the Voice

Perhaps the greatest instrument of healing is the human voice. Toning is a generic term to describe the use of the voice for release of pain and stress, and to help align imbalanced portions of the body. Sighing, moaning, groaning, and other sounds we frequently make are all aspects of toning, as are the sounding of different vowels.

Often, a Sound Healing practitioner will make sounds to a client they are working on. Usually, the client is lying on a table during a session. These sounds made can be purely intuitive, coming through the practitioner as they allow themselves to become a conduit for sacred sound. Some practitioners claim to be able to sense or hear trauma that is trapped in the physical body. By repeating these sounds they are able to release the trauma. Some practitioners work with a technique called "Overtoning".

How to Conduct an Overtoning Session

"Overtoning" is a technique in which a Sound Healer will use his or her own voice to scan the physical body of the client and then project vocal harmonics (overtones) into an imbalanced portion of the body (or etheric center) that is found. A practitioner begins by making a siren-like sound, starting at the bottom of the client's feet with a very low sound and continuing up the body, raising in pitch, until a very high sound is created at the client's head. An experienced practitioner of this technique will be able to hear changes in their tone as they do this. The vocal timbre (or tone color created by harmonics in the voice) actually changes when the sound reaches a place of imbalance. The practitioner then proceeds to project this specific harmonic into the area of the body where the imbalance was found. This may be for a few minutes or longer. When the harmonic become less audible or disappears and the tone becomes normalized, the sounding for that area is complete. Frequently, a practitioner will find a number of areas where sounding is needed. A practitioner may conclude the session with discussion of the experience with the client.

This technique, while quite simple, utilizes a combination of listening and sounding. The practitioner is listening for a change in their tone that occurs as a result of their sound interfacing with the energy field of their client. They must be extremely aware of the subtle changes in their sound in order to do this technique most effectively.

Ayurveda

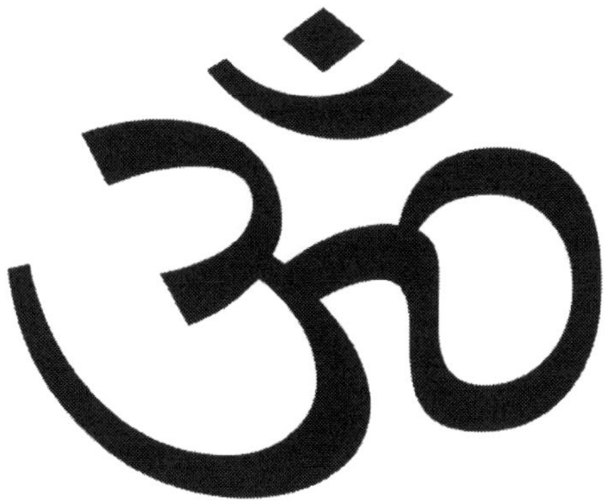

Ayurveda comes to us from the Vedas, the Hindu Scriptures, and demonstrates that true health can be obtained only when physical, emotional, and spiritual wellness are achieved simultaneously. This is the true art of the holistic practitioner.

Ayurveda, which means "science of life", is the traditional healing system of India, which originated over 5,000 years ago. As eastern philosophies are becoming more recognized in the West, so is Ayurveda gaining popularity as a complementary health system.

Ayurveda is the oldest surviving complete medical system in the world. Derived from its ancient Sanskrit roots - 'ayus' (life) and 'ved' (knowledge) – and offering a rich, comprehensive outlook to a healthy life, its origins go back nearly 5000 years. To when it was expounded and practiced by the same spiritual rishis, who laid the foundations of the Vedic civilization in India, by organizing the fundamentals of life into proper systems.

The main source of knowledge in this field therefore remain the Vedas, the divine books of knowledge they propounded, and more specifically the fourth of the series, namely Atharvaveda that dates back to around 1000 BC. Of the few other treatises on Ayurveda that have survived from around the same time, the most famous are Charaka Samhita and the Sushruta Samhita which concentrate on internal medicine and surgery respectively. The Astanga Hridayam is a more concise compilation of earlier texts that was created about a thousand years ago. These between them forming a greater part of the knowledge base on Ayurveda as it is practiced today.

The art of Ayurveda had spread around in the 6th century BC to Tibet, China, Mongolia, Korea and Sri Lanka, carried over by the Buddhist monks traveling to those lands. Although not much of it survives in original form, its effects can be seen in the various new age concepts that have originated from there.

No philosophy has had greater influence on Ayurveda than Sankhaya's philosophy of creation and manifestation. Which professes that behind all creation there is a state of pure existence or awareness, which is beyond time and space, has no beginning or end, and no qualities. Within pure existence, there arises a desire to experience itself, which results in disequilibrium and causes the manifestation of the primordial physical energy. And the two unite to make the "dance of creation" come alive.

Imponderable, indescribable and extremely subtle, this primordial energy – which and all that flows from it existing only in pure existence – is the creative force of all action, a source of form that has qualities. Matter and energy are so closely related that when energy takes form, we tend to think of it in terms of matter only. And much modified, it ultimately leads to the manifestation of our familiar mental and physical worlds.

It also gives rise to cosmic consciousness, which is the universal order that pervades all life. Individual intelligence, as distinct from the everyday intellectual mind, is derived from and is part of this consciousness. It is the inner wisdom, the part of individuality that remains unswayed by the demands of daily life, or by Ahamkara, the sense of `I-ness'.

A Sanskrit word with no exact translation, Ahamkara, is a concept not quite understood by everyone as it is often misleadingly equated to `ego'. Embracing much more than just that, it is in essence that part of 'me' which knows which parts of the universal creation are 'me'. Since 'I' am not separate from the universal consciousness, but 'I' has an identity that differentiates and defines the boundaries of `me'. All creations therefore have Ahamkara, not just human beings.

There arises from Ahamkara a two-fold creation. The first is Satwa, the subjective world, which is able to perceive and manipulate matter. It comprises the subtle body (the mind), the capacity of the five sense organs to hear, feel, see, taste and smell, and for the five organs of action to speak, grasp, move, procreate and excrete. The mind and the subtle organs providing the bridge between the body, the Ahamkara and the inner wisdom, which three together is considered the essential nature of humans.

The second is Tamas, the objective world of the five elements of sound, touch, vision, taste and smell – the five subtle elements that give rise to the dense elements of ether or space, air, fire, water and the earth – from which all matter of the physical world is derived. And it is Rajas, the force or the energy of movement, which brings together parts of these two worlds.

Dense Element	**Subtle Element**	**Sense Organ**	**Motor Organ**	**Function**
Space	Sound	Ears	Vocal Chords	Speaking
Air	Touch	Skin	Hands	Grasping
Fire	Sight	Eyes	Feet	Moving
Water	Taste	Tongue	Genitals	Procreating
Earth	Smell	Nose	Anus	Excreting

It is worth noting that even at the stage of the dense elements the philosophy of creation, which according to Sankaya is now and in the present, without any past and any future, is still dealing with aspects of existence beyond our simple physical realms. The point of contention being that we are the first and foremost spirit experiencing existence. To use Ayurveda in daily life, one has neither to accept nor even understand this philosophy. But it does provide a deeper insight into how Ayurveda works towards betterment of your health.

Ayurveda therefore is not simply a health care system but a form of lifestyle adopted to maintain perfect balance and harmony within the human existence, from the most abstract transcendental values to the most concrete physiological expressions. Based on the premise that life represents an intelligent co-ordination of the Atma (Soul), Mana (Mind), Indriya (Senses) and Sharira (Body). That revolves around the five dense elements that go into the making of the constitution of each individual, called Prakriti. Which in turn is determined by the vital balance of the three physical energies - Vata, Pitta, Kapha and the three mental energies - Satwa, Rajas, Tamas.

Ayurveda thus offers a unique blend of science and philosophy that balances the physical, mental, emotional and spiritual components necessary for holistic health.

According to Ayurveda, the first requirement for healing oneself and others is a clear understanding of the three doshas. The concept of Vata-Pitta-Kapha is unique to Ayurveda and it holds the potential for revolutionizing the healing systems of the West. However, the concept of the three principles and the Sanskrit words, Vata-Pitta-Kapha, are very difficult to translate into Western terms.

Tridosha Concept: Inside the body, there are three doshas which govern the phyico-chemical and physiological activities. These three doshas are Vata (from ether and air), Pitta (from fire and an aspect of water), and Kapha (from water and earth).Individual constitution is acquired at birth and remains constant through life. Through Ayurvedic books, teachers, and courses, one is able to determine one's individual constitution and thereby knowing which direction to take for self-diagnosis purposes.

A balance among the tridosha is necessary for health. For example, the air principle kindles the bodily fire, but water is necessary to control fire, otherwise the bodily fire would burn the tissues. Vata moves Kapha and Pitta, since Kapha and Pitta are immobile. Together, the tridosha governs all metabolic activities; anabolism (Kapha), catabolism (Vata), and metabolism (Pitta). When Vata is out of balance, the metabolism will be disturbed, resulting in excess catabolism, which is the breakdown or deterioration process in the body. When anabolism is greater than catabolism, there is an increased rate of growth and repair of the organs and tissues. Excess Pitta disturbs metabolism, excess Kapha increases the rate of anabolism and excess Vata creates emaciation (catabolism).

In childhood, anabolism and the Kapha elements are predominant, since this is the time of greatest physical growth. In adulthood, metabolism and the element of Pitta are most apparent, because at this stage the body is matured and stable. In old age, catabolism and Vata are most evident, as the body begins to deteriorate.

Characteristics of Body Types

For a better understanding of your Ayurvedic constitution and to cross-check the results of the test, listed below are the principal physical and psychological characteristics of persons with predominantly single dosha constitutions.

Vata

Physically such people are very tall or very short, non- muscular, with thin and bony limbs and have a quick gait with short fast steps. Skin is generally thin, darkish and cool. The hair is thin, dark, coarse and either kinky or curly. The face is usually long and angular, often with an underdeveloped chin. The neck is thin and scrawny. Nose is small and narrow. May be long, crooked or asymmetrical also. Eyes tend to be small, narrow or sunken, dark brown or gray in color, with dull luster. The mouth being small, with thin, narrow or tight lips. Teeth are irregular, protruding, or broken, set in receding gums. And while the voice is weak, low or cracked, speech is fast with interruptions.

Vata people have restless minds and weak memories. They avoid confrontation. Have active and sensitive natures and express themselves through sport and creative pursuits. Likely to be artistic and creative with a good imagination, they will sometimes overindulge in pleasures. And are sexually the most active. Fearful, worrisome and anxious they are into questioning, theorizing and over-analysis. Often dissatisfied with and unable to sustain friendships, they spend money quickly, often on trifles. With light, interrupted sleep of 5-7 hours a day.

Pitta

A moderately well developed physique with muscular limbs and a purposeful, stable gait of medium speed. With a loud, strong voice and precise, convincing speech. The skin is fair, soft, and lustrous, warm, and tends to burn easily in the sun – has freckles, many moles, and a tendency to rashes. And the bodies are hot and sweaty. Characterized by fine and soft, either fair or reddish hair that tends to gray soon. Face is heart-shaped, often with a pointed chin. While the neck is proportionate and of average size. A neat, pointed, and average sized nose matches the average sized eyes that are either light blue, light gray or hazel in color, with an intense luster which get red in summer or after bathing. The mouth being medium, with average lips and medium-sized, yellowish teeth.

Pitas have an intellectual and precise disposition due to a very alert, focused mind. Sharp and knife-like in anger, they are irritable, jealous and aggressive by nature. Discriminating and judgmental, they are articulate, learned and proud. With a developed sense of responsibility, they can take decisions and organize affairs well. Argumentative, but with a sense of humor, their selectively excellent memory makes them fast learners. Moderately passionate in their sexual pursuits, they spend moderately, usually on luxuries.

Kapha

A thick, broad, well-developed frame and large, long limbs go well with a pleasant, deep and resonant voice with low, slow, rhythmic speech. The skin is usually thick, oily, pale or white and cold. Plentiful, thick, wavy, lustrous and generally brown hair is set on a large, rounded and full face. The neck is solid, with a near tree-trunk quality. A large, rounded nose and large, attractive, blue or light brown in color eyes are found in a mouth that is large with big, full lips. Teeth too are big and white and set in strong gums.

Kapha predominated people are calm, steady, considerate - stable, patient personalities they are slow to anger. Not easily provoked, once angry they do not calm down easily. They are honorable, true to their word and avoid lies. Loyal, forgiving and understanding, they can be lethargic, even lazy, if not driven by others. Learning may be slow but memory will be strong. Excellent in logical analysis, they take time before reaching conclusions. Long hours of deep sleep and a strong, enduring sex drive come naturally. While they do save money, it does get spent on food. And there can at times be an element of dullness, given that a Kapha mind is usually too content to seek fresh mental stimulation.

Healthy Eating

In addition to determining the constitution, there are a number of important factors for maintaining good health, related to the diet. This includes foods eaten, time difference between two meals, combination and quantity of foods, cleanliness and proper eating.

- Food should be fresh, hot, tasty and easy to digest.
- There should be at least a four hour difference between any two meals.
- Restrict the number of items in one meal.
- A feeling of heaviness in the stomach indicates improper eating practices.
- Food should be taken only when hungry and according to digestive power.
- Do not eat while watching while angry, emotional, or distracted.
- Do not rush eating or eat too slowly. Chew the food thoroughly.
- Fruits should not be mixed with meals.
- Do not drink with meals or immediately before or after for best digestion.

Proper Sleep

Proper, regulated sleep is very important to maintain the balance of functions in the body. "Early to bed and early to rise" is the key to good health. For an average person, seven hours sleep is sufficient. Excessive sleeping contributes to disease. Regular exercise according to your constitution is extremely beneficial for good health. Yoga is advised as the best type of exercise as it takes care of physical, mental and spiritual health. Yoga and Ayurveda go hand in hand, as the aim of both these sciences is to give perfect health and attain liberation through God consciousness/Universal understanding.

Cleansing

Even after strictly following the above mentioned procedures, some toxins still accumulate in the body as a result of various metabolic activities. It is necessary to eliminate these toxins from the body, as they foster many diseases especially when their quantity increases beyond a certain limit. To maintain efficient physical functioning and to stay healthy, regular elimination of these toxins is required. Ayurveda recommends fasting for one day.

Rejuvenation therapies are prescribed to maintain optimum health and an active lifestyle even in old age. There are many Ayurvedic rejuvenation preparations available, which can be taken according to season and personal constitution.

In daily life, many activities act as rejuvenating tonics in themselves. Good social conduct, morality, good manners and good character are some important factors.

Overall, these guidelines offer an easy way to stay healthy. What's more is that following these guides does not cost anything and helps you lead a more productive life.

Daytime Routine

Waking

The ideal time to wake up is the Brahma Muhürta, which is the two-hour period before sunrise. This is a good time for commencing the day as it gives peace of mind. After waking fully, one should sit quietly in bed for a minute or two and think about the daily activities. This allows one to plan the day. At this stage of the day, there is a greater ability to concentrate, and motivation and determination is at its height. It is especially beneficial to think about or meditate on some good habits or positive changes that one wishes to make.

Washing the face

After getting up, one should wash the face with tepid (room temperature) water. The eyes, nose and mouth should be thoroughly cleaned with water. In extremely cold conditions, or if the person is suffering from a cough, cold or sore throat, it is beneficial to use warm water.

Fill the mouth with water and hold it for 30 seconds. With the water still in the mouth, sprinkle water on open eyes. Spit the water out, close the eyes and massage the eyelids gently with the palms for about one minute. Be gentle and do not apply too much pressure. Look into the mirror to ensure the face, eyes, nose and neck are clean and there are no abnormal signs such as swelling, lumps, insect bites, cuts or bruises.

Evacuation of bowels

Next, drink a glass of water - in winter use warm water. Avoid drinking tea or coffee as they contain caffeine, which increases heat (Pitta) and causes constipation. Going to the toilet to empty the bowels is important in the morning. If there is no urge, drink another glass of water and briefly walk around the room (50 or 100 steps). The water and movement helps in the downward motion of stool and gases, and can stimulate evacuation.

Cleaning the teeth and tongue

In ancient Ayurvedic texts, the use of herbal sticks for oral hygiene purposes is mentioned. Small sticks from various trees, about ten inches long and the thickness of a finger, were used. The stick was crushed by chewing one end of it, to make a brush for cleaning the teeth without hurting the gums. Pungent, astringent or bitter tasting herbs or trees such as neem, Karaïja, and Karvéra were used to make these sticks.

These trees have an antibacterial effect in the oral cavity. The juice secreted from these plants prevents dental diseases and strengthens the gums. In modern times, it is not usually possible to go out and bring home a branch of a tree for brushing teeth! However, Ayurvedic tooth powders or pastes which include parts of certain trees and herbs are often available in health food shops and are good for oral hygiene.

After brushing the teeth, the tongue should also be cleaned. Toxins are often deposited on the tongue in the form of mucus. Advanced Ayurvedic science includes an analysis of the condition, color and location of these mucus deposits to identify corresponding organs that may be imbalanced or diseased. This is a very accurate diagnostic tool for practitioners.

The tongue should be scraped gently three or four times to ensure that the entire area of the tongue is cleaned, including the back. If a tongue scraper is not available, a toothbrush or the index and middle finger can be used to cleanse the deeper end of the tongue.

Chewing cleansing herbs

After cleaning the teeth and tongue one can chew a clove or fresh betel leaf. Chewing herbs not only keeps the mouth fresh and free from odors but also helps in perception of tastes. Mint and Parsley are two good herbs for Westerners for chewing.

Gargling

After chewing the herbs, gargle two or three times with warm water in winter or tepid water in summer. This removes any remaining particles of food or herbs and rinses the mouth. Sesame oil (in moderation) can also be used for gargling. This keeps the jaws and gums strong and assists in the proper chewing of food.

Exercise

Simple exercise may be undertaken for 15 to 20 minutes. Yoga, brisk walking, and muscle stretching are very beneficial in strengthening and coordinating body parts and relaxing mind and muscle.

Oil massage (Abhyanga)

Following exercise, massage with oil (Abhyanga) is undertaken. In the daily routine, one can apply sesame oil or mustard oil. During summer, coconut oil may be used. Olive oil can be substituted if none of these oils are available.

First apply oil to the head and massage gently for a few minutes. Head massage prevents headache, graying of hair, baldness, insomnia, diseases related to the nervous system and impairment of sense organs. Put one or two drops of oil in each ear and use the fingertip to apply oil in the inner portion of nose. Do not put oil in the eyes. Follow this by applying oil to other parts of the body while rubbing gently.

If a busy schedule prevents you from following this procedure everyday, try to do it at least twice a week or every three days. Spend at least 5-10 minutes for Abhyanga and then relax for 5 minutes. On weekends you can spend a longer time massaging (about 20-30 minutes), with 15 minutes relaxation. Oil massage prevents muscle stiffness, dry skin, skin disorders, gives strength to the body, balances the doshas, nourishes the Dhätus and increases Ojas.

Taking a bath

The next activity in the daily routine is taking a bath or shower. Water of normal temperature (not extremely hot or cold), natural soaps and shampoos are best. Warm water can be used in winter. Clean every part of the body thoroughly. Essential oils or aromas may be used according to choice.

After the shower, rub the body with a towel. This opens the pores of the skin, removes oil and old skin and increases blood circulation. It is preferable to take a shower in the morning rather than at night, as it refreshes you after sleep. However, in summer or depending upon the days' activities, a shower in the evening in addition to the morning shower can be revitalizing.

Meditation

Wear clean and comfortable clothes after showering. The clothes should be comfortable, and suitable for the weather. Before eating breakfast, meditating for 5-10 minutes helps clear the mind and relieve tension. Sit in a relaxed position in a quiet and peaceful place. Breathe deeply and methodically. Clear the mind of thoughts and concentrate on the word Aum or a mantra.

A mantra is a word or sequence of words that is repeated. It has spiritual energy and calms the mind, elevates consciousness and produces harmony. A mantra is usually unique to a person and received from a bona-fide spiritual teacher. In case one does not have a personal mantra, the word Aum is spiritually powerful and may be used. The symbol for Aum is, and focusing on it also enhances clarity and peace of mind.

Work

Relax whenever possible between long working sessions. Even sitting back on a chair, closing the eyes and relaxing the mind for 2-3 minutes can make a big difference to peace of mind and the ability to concentrate. If possible, lie down or sit comfortably on a relaxing chair after lunch. Close the eyes and focus on breathing for about five minutes. Deep, abdominal breathing is very relaxing and rejuvenating.

Try to maintain a cooperative, cordial and positive atmosphere at the work place, avoid stress and anxiety. Don't drink too much tea, coffee or cola drinks, or eats salty, processed snacks. This helps prevent over stimulation of the nervous and digestive systems. Walking around briefly or stretching occasionally, if sitting for long periods, can prevent muscle soreness and stiffness, fatigue and eyestrain. Do not work for long periods without taking breaks.

When you return home in the evening, try to relax for at least five minutes. If you have a family, talking or playing with family members will ease the pressure and stress experienced during the day. If you feel tired, take a shower and have a gentle head massage (with or without oil). Wear comfortable clothing.

Try to eat dinner early, if possible before sunset and no later than two hours before bed. The evening meal should consist of food that is light and easily digested. Avoid deep fried, cold foods, dairy products and sweets. Rice and yogurt should be also avoided. The ideal meal consists of salads, boiled or steamed vegetables, vegetable soups and breads.

If reading or writing during the night, adequate light and a chair that supports the back are required. Do not read, write, use computers or watch television for too long. Over indulgence in sex should be avoided. Going to bed early is good, especially if you have a busy or important day coming up the following day. Try to go to sleep by 10 pm or 11 pm at the latest. Brushing the teeth and washing prior to going to bed is hygienic.

The Seasons

The seasons have a natural effect on the tridosha. According to Charaka Saàhitä, the strength of a person is enhanced by adopting suitable diets and routines according to each season. To attain this level of health, one must have knowledge of the qualities of each season and its influence on the tridosha. The doshas accumulate during seasons that share their similar elements or qualities. Once the dosha has accumulated beyond a certain limit, it becomes aggravated and symptoms of this may manifest. Seasons opposite in nature to a dosha pacify it.

For example, Väta is aggravated in dry, windy and cool conditions, such as during autumn. Kapha accumulates in winter, when it is wet and cold and Pitta increases in summers. Aggravated doshas are alleviated by diets and lifestyles that are opposite in nature to the prevailing conditions. So, cooling foods and drinks are beneficial for a Pitta aggravation, and heating foods for a Väta or Kapha aggravation. Seasonal routines to alleviate doshas when they are naturally aggravated are explained below.

Winter
In winter there is a natural accumulation of Kapha and Vata due to the cold and wet weather, so efforts should be made to keep warm and dry. Warm baths, sauna (Svedana), sunbaths and living in an insulated or heated house are beneficial. Heavy, warm and dry clothes should be worn. In winter, massage should mainly consist of dry rubbing. If there is a specific aggravation of Vata, warm oil may be used.

Warm drinks and foods that have a heating effect are preferable to cold or frozen foods and drinks. A light diet is recommended. As the external atmosphere is so cold, the body retains the heat and attempts to preserve it. Therefore, the internal digestive fire or Jaöharägni becomes stronger and is able to metabolize oils, fats and dairy products (yogurt, milk, cheese). Heavier foods can form a larger part of the diet, because they are easier to digest at this time.

Spring

As the heat of the sun increases in spring, accumulated Kapha starts to break up and disperse throughout the body. This weakens the digestive fire/Jaöharägni. and causes many Kapha related disorders. Coughs, sinus problems and hay fever are common during spring.

The heavy and heating diet adopted in winter should be replaced with foods more suitable for warmer weather. Lighter foods that are cooler in nature should be substituted. Sleeping during the day should be avoided as it aggravates Kapha. Regular physical exercise, gargling with warm water (or herbal decoctions) and drinking warm water are beneficial for preventing disease and alleviating symptoms of aggravated Kapha.

Summer

During summer, the sun is at its strongest and the heat increases Pitta. Staying in a cool room or shady place during the day is recommended. Excessive exposure to the heat and sun may cause sunburn, heat or sunstroke. Aromas or essential oils like sandal or rose - that give a cooling effect may be used. One should wear light loose and comfortable clothes.

The diet should mainly consist of cooling sweet foods and drinks. Cucumber, watermelon, fruits, fruit juices (not acidic or citrus varieties), grains, wheat, rice, and milk are ideal. Lots of water (6 to 8 glasses) should be consumed. Sour, pungent and salty foods should be avoided. Hot, spicy, and acidic foods such as chilies, onions, garlic and spices should be also be excluded from the diet or used in small quantities. Tea, coffee, alcohol and smoking should be avoided.

Autumn

In early autumn Pitta is aggravated, and as the conditions become cooler Väta increases. There is a lot of heat in the blood, causing skin irritations like rashes, inflammations, dryness and itching. Massage is good for the skin, and fluid intake should be maintained at 6–8 glasses to a day to cleanse the internal systems. Clothing should provide protection from the wind.

The digestive fire/Jaöharägni. is not very strong, so heavy foods should be minimized in the early part of the season. Sweet light foods are recommended. As it becomes colder and wetter, foods can become heavier and more heating in nature.

Try to avoid sour and acidic foods, as they increase Pitta. Eat vegetables and fruits that are in season with rice, barley and wheat.

Cause of Diseases

All diseases or sicknesses are caused by an imbalance of the tridosha (Vata, Pitta and Kapha). Factors that cause an imbalance of doshas include diet, lifestyle and other activities. To maintain health, it is important to know the factors that create an imbalance of the doshas.

Factors that Increase Vata

Eating large quantities of food that share the light, dry, airy, cold or gas forming Vata elements of air and space. Too much traveling (by any means of transportation).

Staying awake for long hours, late nights or not sleeping adequately.

Excessive exposure to loud or high-pitched sounds.

Watching too much television and over-exposure to computers or any other kind of electrical appliance.

Indulging in excessive sexual activity.

Excessive imagination, overwork or sporting activity.

Taking medicinal, recreational or stimulation drugs.

Aggravation of Vata weakens the nervous system, and can lead to anxiety, depression or emotional instability. Other symptoms caused by aggravation of Vata are joint pains, constipation, dry skin, loss of memory, palpitation, insomnia, muscle stiffness, weight loss, migraine, vertigo and tremors.

Factors that Increase Pitta

Eating large quantities of food that share the pungent, hot, spicy, sour and acidic Pitta elements of fire. This group includes tomatoes, chilies, eggplant, onion, garlic, fried foods, citrus fruits, pineapple, sauces, pickled foods, mustard and vinegar.

Short temper or Eating while angry.

Exposure to heat and sun.

Drinking excessive tea, coffee or alcohol or smoking.

Engaging in competitive activities.

Some of the symptoms caused by excess Pitta are hyperacidity, skin diseases, burning sensations, fever, infections, ulcers and liver disorders.

Factors that Increase Kapha

Eating foods that share the heavy, dense, sweet, oily and moist Kapha elements of water and earth. Foods in this group include meat, dairy products, nuts, avocado, banana, melons, pasta, rice, cakes, breads, custards and puddings.

Overeating.

Eating while sad or grieving.

Sedentary lifestyle or minimal activity.

Sleeping too much, or sleeping during the day.

Symptoms of excess Kapha include asthma, cough, cold, congestion in the chest, and obesity.

Diet

Since diet, along with daily habits, is crucial to the health of an individual, it must be made clear at the outset that there is no standard ideal diet for all people in general. The various factors that need to be kept in mind while working out the ideal diet for each person, which will be distinctly different based on the person's specific constitutional characteristics, are as listed below:

- The natural qualities of each food.
- How those natural qualities can get altered.
- The effects of combining foods – proper and unacceptable combinations.

- The quantity of food intake.
- Individual differences in food intake.
- The places & climate where the food is grown prepared and consumed.
- The effects of the seasons and time of day.
- Avoidance of artificial flavors, chemicals, preservatives and colors.

Diet Composition

One other factor that has remained a matter of great debate worldwide over the ages has been the vegetarianism vs. non-vegetarianism controversy. Initially it was common belief that non-vegetarian diet is superior in that it is full of energetic ingredients and thus provides more strength and stamina. But now it has been scientifically established that vegetarian diet is more natural and useful to human nature.

Non-vegetarian diet contains cholesterol saturated fatty acids that are the root cause of diseases as coronary heart problems, cerebro-vascular accidents (strokes), eye disorders & high blood pressure. With only about 60% of its contents useful for human body, the rest 40% contains harmful toxins. In addition, such diet is usually heavy for the stomach and produces acidity, which in turn can cause problems in the gastrointestinal system.

Another significantly important difference between the two is that fruits & vegetables (cereals and grains, legumes, seedy fruits, citrus fruits, carrot, cabbage, celery, green leafy vegetables, apples, melons, peaches, pears etc.) are rich in dietary fibers that reduces incidence of coronary heart diseases, cancer of intestinal tract, piles, obesity, diabetes, constipation, hiatus hernia, diverticulitis, irritable bowel syndrome, dental caries and gallstones.

Also many disease causing organisms are transmitted through and thrive in animal protein – serious ailments as Encephalopathy and Mad Cow diseases are caused by Bovine Spongi. Similarly the Salmonella Typhimurium bacteria can be passed on through consumed eggs, causing diseases like pneumonia, bronchitis, and typhoid.

Given that the body of non-vegetarian animals contains 10 times more amount of hydrochloric acid than that of vegetarian ones, and that the human body should not be having such a high concentration of hydrochloric acid, it is reasonable to assume that the fact human body is basically meant for a vegetarian diet.

Food for Your Body Type

Food for Vata
- almonds, coconut, peanuts, pine nuts, sesame seeds, and pistachio
- beets and sweet potatoes
- figs, mango, honeydew melon,
-wheat, rye, oats, rice
-eggs, fish, meat,

Food for Pitta
- butter, buttermilk, coconut(fresh), ice-cream, panir
- bitter melon, cucumber, radishes, spinach, squash, zucchini, pumpkin
- grapefruit, lime, lychee, oranges, peaches, pomegranate
- wheat, rice oats, millet

Food for Kapha
- walnuts, dates, honey
- lentils, most beans, dried peas
- Eggplant, spinach, mint, mustard greens, onions
- sour grapefruit, grapes, pears, apples
- black pepper, anise, cinnamon, ginger powder, pickles, red pepper, fenugreek
- barley, corn, millet, buckwheat, rye

Detoxification

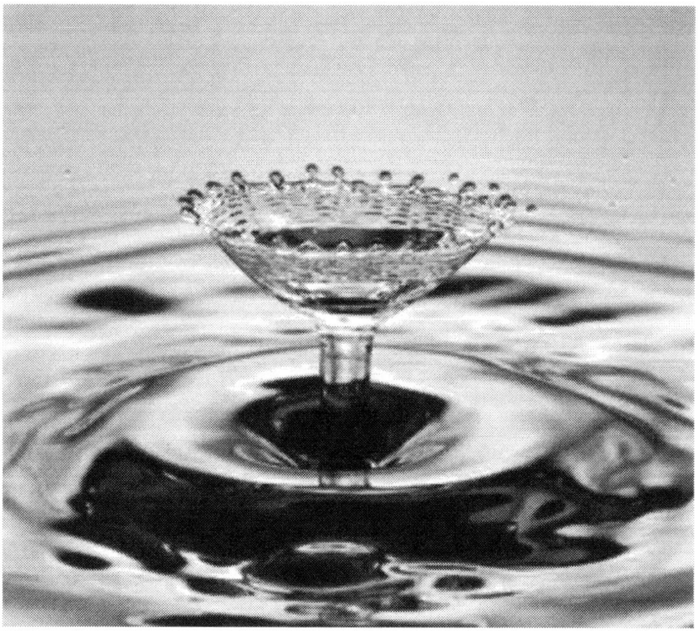

Introduction

There is little doubt that our environment is polluted with toxins and harmful substances. The concepts of internal cleansing and detoxification have been around for centuries. Detoxification of the body refers to the cleansing of the bowels, kidneys, lungs, the liver and the blood since these are the organs involved in the detoxification of chemicals and toxins from the body.

Addictions

So many problems in our Western society come from excessive use of foods and drugs. Abuses and addictions touch almost every person's life. This chapter deals with many of the dietary and substance abuses and ways to heal them.

To begin with, we must ask ourselves--as I suggest to people in their initial medical visit to my clinic--is there anything that we do every day that we would be aware of missing if we would not do it? If so, this activity is a habit or addiction. Of course, there are positive habits. Yet there are many others that may negatively interact with life and health, and can lead to a variety of problems--physically, mentally, and emotionally.

Common addictions in our culture include sugar, various drugs, both pharmaceutical and recreational, caffeine, alcohol, and nicotine. Most adults have problems with one or more of these "drugs," and may even be aware of their habit/addictions and would like to change them, but they don't, can't, or won't for various reasons. In this day and age, we also must be aware of techno-traps, including TV, phone, computers, VCR, FAX, microwaves, and transportation.

Toxins

A toxin is defined as any compound that has a detrimental effect on cell function or structure. Toxins can damage the body in an insidious and cumulative way. Once the internal detoxification system becomes overloaded, toxic metabolites begin to accumulate. We also become progressively more sensitive to other chemicals, some of which are normally non-toxic. It is this accumulation of toxins over a period of time than can wreak havoc on our normal metabolic processes thus causing numerous allergies and addictions.

Toxins include industrial chemicals and their by-products, pesticides, additives in our foods, heavy metals, anesthetics, drugs, environmental hormones, and secondary smoke. More than two million synthetic substances have been identified and 25,000 new toxins are added each year. About 30,000 are produced on a commercial scale.

Do You Need Detoxification?

Most of us cannot escape to a safe haven, free from toxins and pollutants. The air that we breathe is polluted, the water that we drink is full of chlorine, the clothing we wear is made of artificial fabrics and chemicals, the lotions and shampoos that we use all contain chemicals. Once these chemicals are inside us, we can never fully eliminate them unless we undergo a detoxification process. As a result, most of us need some form of detoxification. It is one of the best ways to remain healthy in a polluted and toxic environment.

Our bodies are clearly designed to be self-cleansing and self-healing. The internal detoxification process is an automatic daily procedure of the major detoxification organs. In the past, detoxification was for reformed alcoholics and drugs addicts, people with severe allergies, cancer patients. Nowadays it is adopted by healthy individuals to maintain their body systems in pristine condition.

A weekly, monthly or even quarterly detoxification program can make a big difference in optimizing the bodily functions. In fact, it might even help prevent chronic diseases such as cancer, diabetes, chronic fatigue and arthritis.

Signs that Detoxification is Needed

- If you have unexplained headaches or back pain
- If you have joint pain or arthritis
- If your memory is failing
- If you are depressed or lack energy
- If you have brittle nails and hair
- If you have abnormal body odor, coated tongue or bad breath
- If you have an unexplained weight gain
- If you have psoriasis
- If you have frequent allergies
- If you have a history of heavy alcohol use
- If you have a history of natural and synthetic steroid hormone use.
- If you have an exposure to cleaning solvents, pesticides, and certain drugs

Benefits of Detoxification

1. Digestive tract is cleansed of accumulated waste and fermenting bacteria.
2. System purification occurs that is not possible during regular eating patterns
3. Mental clarity is enhanced as chemical and food additive overload is reduced
4. Reduced dependency on habit forming substances
5. Stomach size is returned to normal as bad eating habits can be stopped
6. Hormonal system is enhanced which is especially true for growth hormone
7. Immune system is stimulated.

Types of Toxins

For the sake of our discussion, we will be discussing the following categories of toxins:

A. Heavy metal toxins
B. Spiritual/Emotional Toxins
C. Specific Substance Detoxification

Heavy Metal Toxins

Lead, mercury, cadmium, arsenic, nickel, and aluminum are included in this category. These metals tend to accumulate in the brain, kidneys and immune system.

Up to 25 percent of the US population suffers from heavy metal poisoning especially from lead, mercury, and aluminum. Over 600,000 tons of lead is released into the atmosphere from industrial processes and leaded gasoline. The toxins could then either be inhaled or ingested after being deposited on food crops, fresh water and soil. Other common sources of heavy metals include lead from pesticides sprays and cooking utensils; cadmium and lead from cigarette smoke; mercury from dental fillings, contaminated fish, and aluminum from antacids, cookware, and soda cans.

Heavy metal toxicity has been linked to several diseases including Alzheimer's Disease, Parkinson's Disease and severe neurological disorders.

Hair mineral analysis is a convenient but often unreliable screening test. The most accurate measurement is by blood analysis of actual toxin levels within the red blood cells. Many toxic metals have a tendency to accumulate inside the cell where most of the damage is done. Serum toxic metal levels do not correlate well with intracellular toxic metal levels.

The early signs of heavy metal poisoning are vague or often attributed to other diseases. The early symptoms of heavy metal poisoning include headaches, fatigue, muscle pain, indigestion, tremors, constipation, anemia, indigestion and tremors. Mild toxicity symptoms include impaired memory and distorted thinking ability. Severe toxicity can lead to death.

Solution: Chelation therapy using high potency multiple-vitamin-and mineral supplement, vitamin C and B complex, sulfur containing amino acids (methionine, cysteine, and taurine), and high sulfur-content foods such as garlic, onion, eggs, water-soluble fibers such as guar gum, oat bran, pectin and psyllium seed. If possible, remove all mercury fillings and consult a holistic dentist for more natural options.

Energetic/Emotional Toxins

Just as the body can experience a build-up of chemicals, sludge, and undigested food, it too can and will accumulate old emotions and experiences. Such examples of energetic toxins are unresolved conflict with family, poor self-image, lifepath uncertainty, and abuse/neglect issues. While this might be the first time you have heard of this form of toxin, it is in fact a complete field of holistic healing onto itself. Any event or emotion, if traumatic enough, can create a long term impact on your health and well-being.

Spiritual and emotional issues, if not identified and confronted, can manifest as illness and dis-ease. Often, when recovery is not experienced after consulting with a physician or competent healthcare provider, it is wise to visit a holistic or spiritual healer for a session. He or she has been trained to identify and balance the energy pathways of the body. While diet, exercise, and other detoxification techniques are beneficial, the best way to remove energetic and emotional toxins is through energy therapies such as Reiki, therapeutic touch, massage, or similar modalities, proper mind set, and personal and spiritual coaching.

Specific Substance Detoxification

There are a number of foods and substances we consume on a regular basis that leave their residue. Often, we are well aware we need to reduce or eliminate their consumption, but their presence in the body is addictive in nature. When they leave the body and are not replenished, often painful symptoms, anxiety, nausea, sweating, and other withdrawal effects are experienced. Any substance that you have difficulty removing from your life has become addictive, and addictions are damaging to mind and body.

Candida/Yeast

Candida Albicans is a yeast infection that begins in the digestive system and little by little spreads to other parts of the body. It is a strong, invasive parasite that attaches itself to the intestinal wall and can become a permanent resident of your internal organs. It is causing numerous health problems and discomfort for over 30 million men and women every day and it is estimated that nearly everyone has or will eventually have a moderate to serious Candida condition in their lives. I personally battled for over two years with Candida, and my husband has been hospitalized, debilitated, and was disabled from working for nearly 12 months due to a severe systematic yeast infection.

A yeast cell produces over 75 known toxic substances that poison the human body. These toxins contaminate the tissues, weakens the immune system, the glands, the kidneys, bladder, lungs, liver and especially the brain and nervous system. Candida yeast can become so massive and invasive that is enters the FUNGAL form where it provides very long, root-like structures that penetrate the mucous lining of the gastrointestinal wall. This penetration breaks down the protective barrier between the intestinal tract and bloodstream, allowing many foreign and toxic substances to enter and pollute the body systemically. As a result, proteins and other food wastes that are not completely digested or eliminated can assault the immune system and cause tremendous allergic reactions, fatigue and many other health problems. It also allows the Candida itself and bacteria to enter the bloodstream, from which it may find its way to other tissues, resulting in far-ranging effects such as soreness of the joints, chest pain, sinus and skin problems, etc. To make matters worse, Candida may be sexually encouraged from one person to another. Candida creates chaos in the intestines and diseases of which the doctors have little or no answer. In fact, there is no blood test for Candida.

Common Symptoms of Candida Overgrowth

Gastrointestinal Tract:
Chronic heartburn, gastritis, colitis, distention and bloating, gas, constipation, diarrhea.

Central Nervous System:
Depression, headaches, lethargy, agitation, hyperirritability, memory loss, inability to concentrate.

Allergic Symptoms:
Hay fever, sinusitis, earaches, hives, asthma, food and chemical sensitivities

Genitourinary Tract:
Yeast vaginitis, menstrual irregularities, cramping, endometriosis, cystitis, urethritis, and kidney and bladder infections.

Generalized Symptoms:
Fatigue, migrating joint pain and stiffness, cold hands and feet, increased body hair, numbness and tingling, food cravings, loss of libido.

Candida Detox Diet

Now that you have made the commitment to deal with your yeast problems, you're going to find that this diet brings relief but only if you adhere to it closely. When you begin your yeast diet, there are two ways it can affect you…you may begin to feel better right away.. or if you are full of toxins, you may feel worse for a few days before you notice improvement. Either way is the right way for you. As you begin to feel better you may decide that it won't hurt to cheat a little here and there. And it may not. But it may. This is where you come in because only you know how you truly feel. And after you cheat, if you find that you feel awful, you will at least know what it is that made you this way. It all comes back to being responsible for yourself.

List of Foods to Avoid Entirely

Sugar -- It is best to eliminate all forms of refined sugar, as it feeds the yeast and encourages its growth. These foods include: white sugar, brown sugar, honey, maple syrup, corn syrup, maple sugar, molasses. Read labels carefully. The hidden sugars to watch for include: sucrose, fructose, maltose, lactose, glycogen, glucose, mannitol, sorbitol, galactose, monosaccharides, polysaccharides.

Fruit -- Fruit contain natural sugars that support the growth of yeast. The following foods should be eliminated:

Yeast, including brewer's yeast and nutritional yeast

Foods Containing Gluten- These include wheat, barley, and rye

Vinegar and foods made with vinegar

Mushrooms

Dairy products, especially cheese

Supplements that May Help Candida

Before taking any supplements, please consult a healthcare provider

Olive Leaf Extract

Garlic

Pau D'Arco

Colloidal Silver

Caprylic Acid

There are also many brands of supplements out there that are herbal and vitamin blends designed to fight yeast, and are available at most local vitamin shops.

Sugar Detoxification

Its common knowledge that sugar is not beneficial to health, and yet most people find that they simply can't eliminate it from their diet. I get asked all the time—can people get addicted to sugar? And the answer is YES. People can get addicted to sugar, sweet foods, and white-flour products (which your body responds to as if they were sugars). This addiction is physiological and affects the same biochemical systems in your body that are affected by addictive drugs like morphine and heroin.

You can actually get "high" on sugar. Eating it can make you feel euphoric immediately. If you don't have your regular sugar "fix," you can experience withdrawal symptoms, such as irritability, headaches, and other flu-like symptoms. Your body can become physiologically dependent upon the effect the sugars have on you.

Your body has a special biochemistry. As a result, you have a different response to sugar than a person with a normal biochemistry. Your heart sings at the sight of a newly opened box of chocolates. Your molecules jump to attention when you get a whiff of bread fresh from the oven. This yearning, however, is not about greed. It is the natural response of a sugar-sensitive person.

After you have worked at shifting to the more complex side of the carbohydrate continuum, and you have been reducing your sugars, you may decide that you are ready to go ahead and eliminate overt sugars altogether.

If you feel you are ready to do this, start by thinking of the process as a detox process. You will be giving up your "drug" and will want to plan a way to minimize your discomfort and maximize your success. Thinking of going off of sugar as "detox" will also help you see that there will be predictable physiological stages and, most important, light at the other end of the tunnel. Going off of sugars doesn't have to be too difficult from a physical standpoint. It may be more difficult from an emotional standpoint. But we will talk about this as we go.

Now it's time to go off sugars. Withdrawal from sugar will feel like withdrawal from a drug. This is because both sugar and narcotics raise our beta-endorphin level and when we stop using them, the brain starts begging for more. The process usually takes five days, with the fourth day being the hardest.

Nicotine

Nicotine is addictive. Most smokers use tobacco regularly because they are addicted to nicotine. It is well documented that most smokers identify tobacco as harmful and express a desire to reduce or stop using it, and nearly 35 million of them make a serious attempt to quit each year. Unfortunately, less than 7 percent of those who try to quit on their own achieve more than 1 year of abstinence; most relapse within a few days of attempting to quit.

Quit Smoking Diet

The vegetarian diet is high in chlorophyllic (green) vegetables and sprouts, grains, fruits, and liquids, such as water, juices, soups, and herbal teas. The raw foods diet is similar, with more seeds and nuts. Eating whole, unsalted sunflower seeds (or carrot or celery sticks) can help replace that hand-to-mouth addiction that is common in smokers; however, we must be careful not to replace nicotine addiction with food addiction.

The diet for detoxification is also low in fat and high in fiber. It is important to keep the energy and bowels moving. The raw foods (and vegetarian) diet helps with both. This includes several salads of leafy greens daily, and some snacks of fruits, vegetables, nuts, or seeds. Some of the high-protein algae, such as spirulina and chlorella, also help during withdrawal and detox.

Supplements

A general "multiple" with additional antioxidant nutrients are part of the smoker's program. The antioxidants help reduce the toxicity of smoke in primary and secondary smokers and also help lessen the free-radical irritation during the detox period. Vitamin E, 400–800 IUs daily, specifically helps stabilize the cell membranes and protects them and the tissue membranes from the free-radical and chemical irritations generated by cigarette smoke. Selenium, as sodium selenite or selenomethionine, at a level of 200–300 mcg., supports vitamin E and also reduces cancer potential, which is so much higher with chronic smoking. Selenium also lessens sensitivity to cadmium. Vitamin A reduces cancer risk and supports tissue health, and beta-carotene specifically protects against lung cancer in smokers. Smoking clearly depletes body vitamin C levels, probably by increasing antioxidant demands and reducing absorption. Therefore, smokers need regular vitamin C intake to help neutralize the toxins. Supplementing 500–2,000 mg. four or five times daily is recommended. (Note: Both vitamin C and niacin are mild acids, which may increase ulcer risk, as well as nicotine elimination and craving in smokers. If these nutrients are used in higher amounts, extra alkaline salts such as the bicarbonates or calcium-magnesium ascorbates, may be used.) Extra zinc, 30–60 mg. a day, like vitamin A, helps protect the tissue and mucous membrane health.

There are many other helpful nutrients needed during smoking and detox. First, we need to support the B vitamins that are more easily depleted in smokers, mainly thiamine (B1), pyridoxine (B6), and cobalamin (B12). The B12 may also help to decrease the cellular damage caused by tars and nicotine. Niacin (B3) helps in opening up the circulation that is constricted with nicotine. It also lowers cholesterol, which may reduce the risk of atherosclerosis. Pantothenic acid may reduce the aging of the skin and support the generally stressful lifestyle. Folic acid should be taken in higher amounts, such as 1–2 mg. daily. Coenzyme Q10 is also helpful in dosages of 30–60 mg. daily. Extra choline may support the brain and memory.

During withdrawal, I suggest taking vitamin C (as a mineral ascorbate to reduce acidity) in amounts of about 1 gram every one or two hours. This may help reduce nicotine cravings. Other nutrients and dietary plans discussed earlier may also be used. The maximum dosages listed in the table at the end of this section can be used for support during withdrawal.

Alcohol Detoxification

Diet and megavitamin therapy may be helpful during withdrawal, detoxification, and recovery from alcoholism. Alcoholics while drinking generally need more supplements than most other people. And during the detox time, they may need even more. This extra support will give a greater chance of recovery than just having psychotherapy. As I just mentioned, attending AA meetings may aid alcoholics greatly.

During the actual withdrawal period, which may last from a few days to a week, the diet can be focused on fluids and the alkaline foods. The appetite is usually not great, and liquids will help in clearing alcohol from the body. Water, diluted fruit and vegetable juices, warm broths and soups, and teas using herbs, such as chamomile, skullcap (a nervine), or valerian root all will serve the needs. Some other herbs that may be helpful during withdrawal are white willow bark to reduce pain and inflammation, ginseng, cayenne, and peppermint. Small amounts of light proteins, such as nonfatty poultry, fish, or even chicken soup, will provide more nourishment. Amino acid powder can also be supportive. Up to 2-3 grams of L-tryptophan can be taken for sleep. L-glutamine, another amino acid, has been shown to reduce cravings for alcohol and sugar, and is used in many detox clinics.

Alcohol detoxification continues for at least several weeks after the withdrawal period. During this recovery time, the body will eliminate alcohol, its by-products, and other toxins and begin breaking down some of the fat that may have been stored during alcohol abuse. General supportive and balanced nourishment with a low-fat, moderate protein, basic complex carbohydrate diet is recommended. Since alcoholics often have blood sugar problems, basic hypoglycemic principles should be followed. These include avoiding sugars and refined foods, soft drinks, candy, and so on; small amounts of fruits and fruit juices may be tolerated. Regular eating every few hours is recommended. Small meals and snacks of protein or complex carbohydrate, including whole grains, pasta, potatoes, squashes, legumes, and other vegetables, can be the basic diet. Proteins such as soy products, eggs, fish, or poultry can also be added, but the basic aim is to maintain an alkaline diet, so the primary focus initially during withdrawal should be on vegetables and fruit.

Water should be drunk throughout the day as well; chamomile or peppermint teas can also be used. All alcoholic beverages should, of course, be eliminated. Foods containing potentially damaging fats, including fried foods, chips, burgers, hot dogs, fast foods, and ice cream should also be avoided. These foods are all congesting and more acid-forming as well. Caffeine and cigarette smoking are best minimized. Many recovering alcoholics take in large amounts of coffee and smoke intensely, as can be clearly seen at AA meetings. This is not recommended at all. These habits suggest a need for stronger psychological support to become generally less addictive. Luckily though, in recent years there is a strong faction for nonsmoking AA meetings, and this is a big plus.

During detoxification from alcohol (usually from other substances, too), many other important nutrients besides diet can be added. Amino acids can be used, including L-tryptophan for sleep. Calcium and magnesium supplements taken at night may also aid sleep, as may valerian root capsules. L-glutamine is an amino acid that generates glutamic acid, and this can get directly into the brain and be used for fuel. Glutamine is naturally found in liver, meats, dairy foods, and cabbage. It can diminish the craving for alcohol and sugar (chromium may also help with sugar cravings). A dosage of 500-1,000 mg. three times daily between or before meals is suggested, as capsules or as L-glutamine powder, taken before or after meals and before bed.

A basic "multiple" along with antioxidant nutrients can be employed during detoxification from alcohol. Extra minerals, such as zinc, iron, calcium, and magnesium, can be taken to replace those lost during alcohol abuse. Higher levels of niacin, even up to several grams, along with 5-10 grams of vitamin C daily, have been used with some success in alcohol withdrawal and detox. A more modest level of C would be 500-1,000 mg. taken four to six times daily.

Other detoxifying nutrients include additional fiber, which helps to bind toxins in the bowel and improve elimination. Choline and inositol, about 500 mg. each three times daily, will improve fat digestion and utilization. Lemon water with a couple of teaspoons of olive oil and a quarter teaspoon or capsule of cayenne pepper will help detoxify the liver. Taking fiber along with oil decreases the oil absorption, but olive oil alone is thought to be nourishing to the liver and helpful in clearing chemical toxins. Cold-pressed olive oil is part of many natural liver therapies. Goldenseal root powder, one or two capsules twice daily, is also helpful for toning and clearing the liver. Parsley tea improves kidney elimination and cleansing of the blood. The amino acid L-cysteine is another helpful detoxicant for the liver, blood, and colon.

Caffeine Detox

Anyone with regular caffeine intake should truly consider withdrawing from their habit until they can reach a state of occasional use and enjoyment. For caffeine detoxification, it is important to support ourselves nutritionally while we eliminate or reduce our intake. If we are clearly addicted to caffeine products or if we become pregnant, we should quit totally. Breaking the habit by tapering down or going "cold turkey" will be better handled with a good diet and adrenal support.

An alkaline diet is helpful during detoxification. Fruits can be used as snacks; vegetable salads, soups, greens, seaweed, corn, some whole grains, sprouts, soy products, and some nuts and seeds are the basis of this high-nutrient diet. A decrease in acid foods, such as meats, sugar (avoiding sugar may really help minimize caffeine withdrawal), and refined flours, and avoiding overuse of baked goods, even whole grain products, and nuts and seeds are good ideas. Drinking at least six to eight glasses of filtered water and sipping on some mineral waters can help replace the coffee habit. Often, some baking soda or, even better, potassium bicarbonate tablets, will help make us more alkaline and reduce withdrawal symptoms.

Vitamin C supplementation also helps during withdrawal and supports the adrenals. As an anti-stress program, several grams or more of vitamin C can be taken over the course of the day, preferably in a buffered form, along with certain minerals such as potassium, calcium, magnesium, and zinc, all of which often need to be supplemented. B complex vitamins with extra pantothenic acid (250 mg. four times daily) along with 500 mg. of vitamin C every two hours can be helpful in withdrawal.

With general coffee usage, we need to support the commonly depleted nutrients. These include thiamine (B1), riboflavin (B2), pyridoxine (B6), vitamin C, potassium, magnesium, and probably zinc, iron, calcium, and the trace minerals. Sometimes additional amino acids are helpful in balancing our energy level during use or withdrawal from caffeine. Water intake and additional fiber, even on top of a high-fiber diet, will help support the bowel function, which can slow down during caffeine withdrawal.

For caffeine detoxification, it is definitely easier to detox over a week or two to avoid significant headaches and other symptoms, although some regular users can stop fairly easily without many problems. Drinking grain-coffee blends, diluted or smaller amounts of regular coffee, or decaffeinated coffee (only if it is water processed) is a good way to reduce caffeine intake. Some people can substitute tea, which has less caffeine, and taper off of that more easily.

If headaches occur during detoxification, some mild pain relievers can be used for a few days, but not much longer. Increased water intake, vitamin C and mineral support, an alkaline diet, and white willow bark herb tablets, which contain a natural salicylate, may also ease withdrawal.

Drug Detoxification

Any of the thousands of prescription and over-the-counter (OTC) drugs currently available and in common use can be toxic, especially when too much is used or when they are used for too long. Aspirin and other anti-inflammatory and pain-relieving drugs, tranquilizers, and anti-depressants are all in very common use.

Using sleeping pills, tranquilizers, and antidepressants is another way to deal with life's frustrations and challenges. Valium has been a very popular drug, the most popular for a few years, but new drugs keep entering the race, and Ativan, Xanax,

Halcion, and others are now also very popular. Barbiturates are less common now; they used to be the main sedatives but now are probably more frequently used on the street. All these drugs that slow us down, mainly by depressing our nervous system, act like alcohol, so review the Alcohol Detoxification program along with this one if these drugs are an interest or problem.

Stimulants, such as the amphetamines and cocaine, are on the opposite end of the spectrum from sedatives. They are very stimulating but also cause dramatic fluctuations in energy. They excite the nervous system and cause euphoria or irritability with resultant loss of appetite, hypersensitivity, and insomnia, usually followed by fatigue and depression. As with the narcotics, amphetamine withdrawal and detoxification often require professional assistance, although some people manage to do it on their own. The stimulant drugs in general are more deadly than most others, including narcotics, so it is very important to eliminate them if we want to live long and healthy lives.

A general detox program for a pharmaceutical or OTC drug involves first familiarizing yourself with its effects, side effects, addiction potential, and withdrawal symptoms (preferably, we do this before we use it).

Some drugs are dangerous to stop. Going "cold turkey" from sedatives, stimulants, and narcotics can have serious consequences, including seizures. Tranquilizers may be needed to get us through the withdrawal phase. Overall, a plan should be made with the help of a professional, such as consulting a medical doctor of psychologist to help in withdrawal.

Cocaine

Cocaine is extremely addicting, both psychologically and physically (over time of course, not with one try; however, its withdrawal can be seen after any usage) and is very costly, often causing financial ruin to the addicted and his or her family. Cocaine withdrawal can be very difficult, particularly psychologically (the opiates, for example, seem to be more physically addicting).

For cocaine detoxification, as with healing from any drug, first we must acknowledge that we have a problem and decide to do something about it. We should get rid of all the drugs and paraphernalia and drop friends and associates that are tied to our drug problem. We can seek (and accept) the support of our spouse, friends, or relatives if we are comfortable with that. For actual withdrawal, we should prepare for symptoms with the aforementioned nutrients and the support of a professional. Tranquilizer drugs may be needed for a few days or longer, but these must be handled sensitively, as one addiction can easily replace another. Psychological counseling and/or a support group can help prevent any new addictions.

Marijuana

Cannabis sativa (and indica), or marijuana, is the most commonly used illegal drug in the Western world. In the United States, it has become a megabusiness. For many years, it was thought to be fairly innocuous, but now most medical authorities believe that marijuana is not a harmless drug at all and that with regular use it can lead to many problems, both acute and chronic.

For marijuana detoxification, as with other drugs, we must first decide that it is a problem and plan to stop, seeking support from companions. Avoid "pothead" friends and get rid of the "stuff" and associated paraphernalia. The tetrahydrocannabinol (THC), marijuana's active ingredient, gets stored in the body fat and liver, so as we detox, some of the withdrawal symptoms or flashbacks may surface, but usually they are pretty mild. With exercise, sweats, or weight loss, the fat will release toxins, but this is also helpful for a faster clearing. It is wise with marijuana withdrawal to avoid other drugs, tranquilizers, and cigarette smoke and to know and believe that we can stop it. As with alcohol and other only mildly toxic drugs, people seem to be able to use it occasionally for social or relaxation reasons, but when it becomes a regular habit, it is wise to avoid it completely.

Detoxification Protocol

3 Principals of any detoxification program

Cleansing

Rebuilding

Maintenance

Cleansing of the body system is done internally through fasting and externally through thorough skin cleansing. Enemas can also be used but are normally reserved for cases where intense cleansing is required, as is often the case in using detoxification as a way to treat cancer.

Fasting Cleanse

This is best accomplished by simple fasting. Dramatic changes can be seen as masses of accumulated waste is expelled as the body rids itself of toxins. Short bouts of headaches, fatigue, body odor, bad breath, diarrhea or mouth sores are commonly accompanied by accelerated excretion. However, digestion usually improves immediately as do many organ and nerve functions.

Cleansing by fasting can last from one day to a week. This depends on the timeframe, the body's requirements, toxic load and the patient's overall heath.

During fasting, the release of toxins is common. This is especially so if you are overloaded with toxins or have a long history of exposure to fat-soluble toxins such as pesticides. Stored toxins in the cells are released into our system during fasting. For example, the pesticide DDT has been shown to be mobilized during a fast and may reach blood levels toxic to the nervous system. You may actually feel worse before feeling better.

The best way to proceed is to start slow with a three-day vegetable juice fast. Longer fasts require strict medical supervision while the shorter fast can usually be conducted at home. It is essential to consult a physician especially if you have medical conditions such as diabetes that may be worsened during a fast.

Prepare for fasting on the day before with fresh fruits and vegetables on the last meal. During the fast, take a high potency multiple-vitamin-and-mineral formula to provide general support. Take 1000 mg of vitamin C three times a day and one to two tablespoons of a fiber supplement at night before sleep. If you are particularly overloaded with toxins, consume 70 to 210 mg of silymarin thrice a day.

Exercise is not usually encouraged while fasting to conserve energy. It is also important to rest during a fast. A nap or two during the day is recommended. Less sleep will be needed at night since daytime activity is lower. During a fast, the body temperature usually falls. Blood pressure, pulse and respiration rates will also drop to reflect a slow down of the body's metabolic rate. It is therefore important to stay warm. More rest is encouraged to yield better results as energy can then be directed towards healing instead of other bodily functions. When it comes to breaking your fast, it is important to re-introduce solid foods gradually by limiting portions. It is a good idea to eat slowly and chew thoroughly at room temperature. Do not overeat.

Juice Fasting

An excellent way to develop good health and toxin cleansing is by juice fasting. This is because juices, without their pulp (fiber), contain excellent sources of vitamins, minerals and enzymes. Vegetable juices are preferred over fruit as one is able to drink more vegetable juice than they are able to eat. For example, one can readily drink the juice of several heads of lettuce at one go but may not be able to consume the same amount of lettuce as a whole. Juices also contain good sources of antioxidants and enzymes needed for toxin cleansing and excretion. At the same time, they are easy to digest and thus can help to eradicate digestive problems. As a result, drinking juices allows the body to receive plenty of nutrients with minimal digestive action needed. Moreover, fasting on mono-juices allows the body to have sufficient time to process these juices and valuable digestive enzymes can be preserved. During fasting, a sense of well-being, renewed energy, clearer thoughts and a cleaner body system can be resulted.

Vegetable Juicing Program

Fruit juices are very different from vegetable juices. Fruit juices should be avoided as the high sugar content of fruit juices raises the blood sugar and insulin levels. This can lead to insulin resistance and ultimately diabetes in the long run.

Although carrots and beets are vegetables, they are high in sugar content and can raise the blood sugar level much like fruits. Vegetable juicing is not easy. Start slowly by drinking only one or two ounces and finally up to 12 ounces each time. There should be no waves of nausea or belching.

Vegetable juices are not as pleasant-tasting as fruit juices. The beginner should begin by gulping the juice as this is probably the best way to get started. This process will ensure that the juice is in minimal contact with the taste buds.

Take some vegetables before, during or after the juicing. The chewing motion will stimulate gastric juice secretion and aid digestion. It is also important to do some chewing during juicing. As vegetable juicing is not a natural phenomenon in modern day society, the body will need some time to adapt. It is important to pay heed to your body's signals on which vegetable juices to consume and which types to continue in small amounts.

The pulp is one of the best parts of the juice although its palatability leaves much to be desired. It adds bulk and fiber to your diet and helps bowel movements. Try mixing 10 percent of the pulp back into the juice and slowly increase the amount in accordance with your tolerance level. Very few people can consume all the pulp juice as it is quite thick and would look like a bowl of porridge instead of a glass of juice.

All vegetable juices should be consumed immediately. Vegetable juice is one of the most perishable foods. Do not keep for more than 24 hours. Storage is tricky. Oxidation should be prevented. If you have to keep the juice, put it in a glass jar with an airtight lid and fill it to the brim to minimize air space. The oxygen in the air (remember air contains 20 per cent oxygen) will "oxidize" and damage the juice. Wrap the jar with aluminum foil to block out all light, which will also damage the juice and then store it in the refrigerator. The juice should be taken out of the refrigerator 30 minutes prior to consumption, as it should ideally be consumed at room temperature.

The beginner should start with celery, fennel (anise) and cucumbers. These vegetables may not be the most nutritious but at least they are more tolerable and palatable than others. Once the beginner is used to the taste of vegetable juices, other recommended vegetables include spinach, cabbage, bok choy, endive and lettuce. Herbs can also be added to juices such as parsley and cilantro.

The advanced juicer should try Collard Greens, Dandelion Greens and Mustard Greens as these vegetables are very beneficial. These greens are quite bitter tasting, but they are good for you. To make your juice more palatable, you can also add small quantities of carrots and beets. These vegetables are relatively high in sugar content compared to their green leafy counterparts. Coconut is another option to improve the taste of vegetable juices. They are also a good source of fat to balance the meal.

Beginner Juice Recipe

- CARROT JUICE. High in antioxidant: beta-carotene and enzymes.
- CELERY JUICE. High in calcium, and promotes tissue flexibility.
- BEET JUICE. Nourishes the liver and aids in liver function.
- CABBAGE JUICE. High in Vitamin C and anti-cancer properties

Blend the above vegetables in a juicer and consume it immediately. Beets and carrots are higher in calorie content in comparison with cabbage and celery. Do not consume carrot and beet juices if you have a history of sugar imbalance.

Simple 24 Hour Juice Fasting Detoxification Program

Juice fasting enables the digestive system to rest and also speeds up the growth of new cells, which in turn promotes healing. A person on a juice fast should abstain from solid foods and drink fruit and vegetable juices, water and herbal teas throughout the day. While vegetable juices are superior to fruit juices on a day-to-day basis, fruit juices are often recommended in part during a fasting program. Calorie from the sugar in the fruit juice is needed to avoid hypoglycemia.. The fasting period varies from person to person although every half-hour to an hour is the norm. Frequent juicing will supply the body with adequate amounts of energy throughout the day. Drink at least four 8 to 12 glasses of water every day during the fast. Avoid coffee, bottled, canned or frozen juice (primarily sugar) and soft drinks. Unsweetened herbal teas are acceptable.

The night before: consume a simple dinner with a green leafy salad. Dry brush your skin before you go to bed to open your pores for the night's cleansing eliminations.

On rising: one glass of two freshly squeezed lemon juice. One tablespoon of maple syrup and 8-oz of pure water at room temperature (filtered but not distilled) .

Midmorning: one glass of cranberry juice from concentrate to promote bowel movement.

Lunch: one glass of fresh apple juice.

Mid-afternoon: one cup of herbal tea.

Dinner: One glass of papaya /pineapple juice to enhance enzyme production or another glass of apple juice.

Before bed: one cup of mint tea, miso soup or hot water for relaxation.

Next morning: break your fast with fresh fruits and yogurt. Consume light, raw foods during the day and a simple, low fat dinner.

The same plan can be extended over the weekend for a three-day detoxification program.

Skin Cleanse

As our skin is one of the most effective excretion organs, a detoxification program on skin cleansing is essential. When we sweat, heavy metal compounds are eliminated through the skin's pores.

Therefore good skin care is essential to optimum health. Even though chemicalized skin care products such as soaps and shampoos may be cheaper, they are not recommended. When these chemicals are absorbed into our body circulation, they in effect add more "toxins" into our system. Most people fail to understand its ill effects because their liver is able to metabolize the toxins. Yet, there are some environmentally friendly people who experience great differences in their health when they use natural soaps and shampoos.

There are several ways to get rid of toxins through the skin, namely exercise, sauna, skin brushing and detoxification baths, to name a few.

a. Skin Brushing. This helps the skin to remove its outer dead layers and keep the pores open. Besides brushing, one can try toweling off vigorously until the skin is slightly red after bathing. Thus, towels have to be changed regularly as they may contain toxins. For effective skin detoxification, good nutrition is also required. Since our skin is made up of mainly fats, natural high quality fats and oils are needed to keep our skin healthy. Two excellent natural oils are butter and olive oils, which keep the skin in a good condition

b. Sauna and steam baths. These are good ways to remove toxins from the skin and regenerate one's health and energy. The sauna is a good follow-up to dry skin brushing because it "pushes" toxins out through the skin. The main thing to remember with saunas is to limit the time spent. Perspiration is encouraged but do not attempt to remain in a sauna for too long as too much heat can dry the skin which in turn accelerates aging.

c. Detoxification bath. Daily bath using natural soaps is essential. Take care of your skin using only natural oils and natural products. We also need to consider our clothing materials carefully as they can have a tremendous effect on our health. Natural fiber clothing is favored over synthetic fiber as the former can help eliminate toxins. Another skin cleansing method is skin brushing. This is simple and relaxing. Try the following: Use ½ cup of baking soda or use ½ cup of Epsom salt or use ½ cup of sea salt. Soak for 15-20 minutes and then scrub the skin gently with soap on a natural fiber. The water will turn murky and "dirty" within minutes as the heavy metals (aluminum and mercury) are excreted from the skin. Detoxification baths should be done once a week and maintenance once a month.

You might also want to consider a filter for your shower, as most of us will absorb more toxins from bathing or showering than from drinking tap water. Needless to say, swimming in the ocean is a much better option than in a chlorinated swimming pool.

Colon Cleanse

Colon cleansing has been used for 4000 years as a health practice of detoxification. Through this process, the large intestine or colon can be healed, rebuilt and finally restored to its natural size, normal shape and correct function.

It is an alternative to health hydrotherapy that gradually and gently cleanses the colon by flushing with a warm water solution. Colon cleansing is preventive healthcare as there is no better place to begin to rid your body of toxins and contamination which may cause cancer, colitis, digestive disorders, fatigue and obesity.

Some of the common agents used in this stage include flaxseed tea, white oak bark and slippery elm bark. These herbs soothe, lubricate and introduce powerful healing agents directly into the large intestine.

Herbal teas may be taken orally concurrently with colon cleansing. Simple dietary changes have been made by now, such as the addition of water.

Most people think of colon irrigation (enemas) as an uncomfortable experience. It is in fact a very quick and effective way to loosen impacted feces and wash away toxins. It also removes many of the unpleasant symptoms of detoxification. Firstly, a sterile tube is inserted into the rectum and filtered warm water washes around the colon for about 15 minutes. An evacuation tube removes the water thus removing years of accumulated debris and mucus.

If the thought of enema bothers you, consider a colon cleansing diet slowly as follows:

Start with a diet of 50 per cent raw food along with a teaspoonful of linseed (available from health food stores) or two level teaspoonfuls of Metamucil. Such bulking agents are readily available at pharmacies or grocery stores. You can chew the linseed to release the nutrients. Water is an essential element in the cleansing process. Start the day with at least half a pint of water, preferably hot, before breakfast. Aim for two quarts per day while you are cleansing the colon unless this conflicts with advice from your doctor.

Lung and Lymphatic Cleanse

Aerobics exercise, which is widely, associated with cardiovascular health also helps cleanse the lungs. During active and intense exercise, forced expiratory volume of the lung's oxygen exchange capacity is increased and "dead air" normally trapped within the small alveoli of the lungs is expelled in exchange for fresh air. It is important to exercise in non-polluted areas.

Breathing exercises combined with physical activity increase the action of lymphatic cleansing. This can be done when you synchronize your breathing with the movement of your legs and arms. For example, when you are walking or jumping on the trampoline, inhale four times and exhale four times. Move your arms and legs each time you take a small breath. Inhale through your nose and exhale through your nose or mouth.

In addition to exercise, especially walking, the lymph system is effectively cleansed from such activities as dry brushing of the skin, lymph node massage performed by a specially trained therapist, and hot water with lemon juice.

Kidney and Blood Cleanse

To optimize kidney cleaning, one quart of pure filtered water per day for every 50 pounds of body weight is one of the absolute basic foundations for anti-aging. If you are in good health, try drinking 10 to15 glasses of water daily. It is best to limit your intake to filtered or bottled water.

The right kind of water is especially important. Distillation is the process in which water is boiled, evaporated and the vapor condensed. Distilled water is devoid of dissolved minerals and is thus able to actively absorb toxic substances from the body and eliminate them. Taking distilled water during detoxification for a short period of time (less than 4 weeks) helps the body to eliminate unwanted minerals. Once this is accomplished, distilled water consumption should be discontinued.

The ideal water for long term human consumption should be slightly alkaline and contains minerals such as calcium and magnesium. Water filtered through reverse osmosis tends to be neutral and is recommended for long term consumption. Water filtered through a solid charcoal filter is slightly alkaline. Make sure that the filter you choose is of good quality and remove pollutants and parasites such as cryptosporidium. If you do not possess a water filter, bottled water is the next best option. It should however be highlighted that about 25 to 30 percent of the bottled water sold in the United States comes from tap water which could sometimes be untreated.

Rebuilding

The body can only rebuild with the proper raw materials. A diet comprising mainly fresh and simple prepared food is the best option. It should be very low in trans or hydrogenated fat, sugar, caffeine, sugar, diary, and tobacco. Meats should only be consumed in small amounts. Fresh foods that are low in sugar such as vegetables, soy, organic egg, grains, and seeds are encouraged. Deep-water fish in moderate amounts (once or twice a week) is recommended. The anti-aging Mediterranean diet is a good lifelong diet to rebuild your body's defense system through an abundance of antioxidants.

A rebuilding detoxification diet provides nutritional fortification for the body's immune system. While there are many different detoxification approaches available, they differ in their actions and purpose. Some detoxification programs only effect the bowels. Others may cleanse the liver or blood while others may aid the kidneys or the skin in their functions. Conditions that must be considered in the detoxification process are nutrition, water, exercise, rest, sunshine, and fresh air. By combining these detoxification programs into a total anti-aging program, one can effectively regain health to an optimal level and thus look younger in the process. Once detoxification of the body takes place and when the body eliminates toxins, health is restored and vigor is revitalized.

A natural vegetarian diet is the best way to eliminate toxins from the body effectively. This diet provides fiber needed for stimulating good bowel movements and proper amounts of vitamins to nourish the detoxification organs. As most vegetarian diets are eaten raw, they contain a valuable source of enzymes, which cleanse and aid the body in eliminating toxins. In fact, an elimination of meat from the diet for a short period of time enables the detoxification process to be more effective because meat is difficult to digest.

Adopting a healthy eating lifestyle and diet is however easier said than done. There are many people who seek good health and will do their best to improve their diets. However, there are some who are not keen to make any lifestyle changes. They may make a few changes such as drinking more water.

In summary, a rebuilding detoxification diet is essentially a vegetarian diet consisting of whole fruits, green leafy vegetables, legumes, and seeds. Meat and fish are taken sparingly, if at all. Organic eggs are acceptable in reasonable quantities. Food groups are rotated every four days to allow maximum elimination from the body before another quantity of the same food group are ingested.

Maintenance

Keeping your body clean and toxin free is very important after detoxification. A healthy lifestyle should incorporate the five pillars of anti-aging namely exercise, diet, supplementation, stress reduction and hormonal enhancement. This is the best way to maintain your body in a clean and detoxified state.

Detoxification Enhancing Supplements

In addition to cleansing, rebuilding and maintenance, there are four types of supplementations commonly used to enhance the detoxification program.

As detoxification diets may not stimulate the liver, lungs or the kidneys enough, herbal detoxification supplementation is often added. Not only do herbs provide vitamins, minerals and enzymes-essential for good nutrition, they are also useful in helping certain organs when different herbs are combined. Different herbal combinations aid different organs and they could be found in most organic food stores.

Liver is the main detoxification center of the body. Any successful detoxification regiment should include cleansing and protecting the liver. There are a wide variety of plants that exert beneficial effects on liver functions.

The most impressive research has been done on a special extract of milk thistle (Silybum marianum) known as silymarin, a group of flavonoid compounds. These compounds protect the liver from damage and enhance the detoxification process.

Silymarin prevents damage to the liver by acting as an antioxidant. It is much more effective than vitamin E and vitamin C. Numerous research studies have demonstrated its protective effect on the liver. Experimental liver damage in animals is produced by extremely toxic chemicals such as carbon tetrachloride, amanita toxin, galactosamine and praseodymium nitrate. Silymarin has been shown to protect the liver against these toxins. The common dosage for silymarin is 70 to 200 mg one to three times a day.

- Liver: Dandelion, milk thistle, angelica, gentian, parsley, horsetail, chamomile.
- Kidneys: Parsley, dandelion, juniper berries, bladderwrack, kelp.
- Lungs: Mullein, Marshmallow, osha root.

Herbs are found mainly in the form of teas, powders or extracts. Herbal teas can be made and consumed readily throughout the day, as they are mild and gentle. As there are different styles in preparing teas, experimentation may be done until one finds a suitable tea. Herbal ingredients and commonly used ingredients that enhance intestinal motility include: senna leaf, peppermint leaf, stevia leaf, buckthorn bark, damiana leaf, RED peel, chamomile flower, and uva ursi leaf.

It is always good to eat your regular meal fortified with digestive enzymes to enhance breakdown of food in the gastro intestinal tract as a routine practice. After the evening meal, you can begin drinking tea. Start slowly. You should begin by steeping the tea just 2 minutes (in 1-2 cups of water) for the first 3-5 days. As your system adjusts, you may increase steeping to 5 minutes. Most individuals will experience increased bowel movements or slight cramping during the first few days. This is due to the initial cleansing of the body's system and is normal.

Here is an example of a simple herbal cleansing program that can be used in conjunction with a detoxification diet

- Rising: Drink a glass of lemon water or plain water with an additional teaspoon of apple cider vinegar and a teaspoon of blackstrap molasses.
- Morning: Drink a glass of plain water with added psyllium husk powder (a glass of water following that).
- Meals: Have two to three multi-digestive enzymes and liver herbs.
- In between meals: Drink herbal teas to support the liver.

For effective detoxification, herbs should be used in conjunction with the detoxification diet.

Want to Learn More?

Crystal and Gemstone Therapy

Many people use crystals and gems in their holistic practice. If you are interested in using crystals in your practice, you may want to supplement this course with the Gemology Course offered through Reiki Rays Institute.

Chakra Therapy

Chakra Therapy, which was introduced in this book, is a wonderful supplement to your practice, and is highly recommended for those wishing to continue on. It is non-invasive, can be done on any living thing, and is something you can do on yourself regularly. Most professional holistic practitioners include a full chakra balancing as part of a formal session, so learning how to do this will greatly enhance your clients' experience.

Aromatherapy

Aromatherapy is the study of how scents affect mood and induce healing. This is perhaps the best course to supplement all other holistic therapies with, as you do not even need to anoint oils on the client for them to begin to feel the benefits. Essential oils can be applied "neat" (directly onto the feet), rubbed onto your hands, or diffused in the air.

Reflexology

Reflexology is the application of pressure and movement to the feet to effect corresponding parts of the body. Reflexologists know that the feet are a mirror image of the body. By applying one of several techniques and grips, a reflexologist can break up patterns of stress in other parts of the body. Incorporating Reflexology is a standard part of my own Reiki practice and is why amongst many other practitioners in the area, I am in high demand.

Holistic Health Practitioner Certification

This is a wonderful goal for those who are or plan to enter this rewarding field. It is awarded as a special bonus for those who successfully complete 5 related courses on our site. Please inquire about this program if you are interested.

For a full list of courses and programs, go to www.reikiraysinstitute.com

About the Author

Dawn Grey, PhD, ND, is the President and founder of Reiki Rays Institute. She holds a BA, Magna Cum Laude, in English Literature, a Masters and PhD in Natural Health, and a Doctor of Naturopathy (N.D). She has also completed additional post graduate studies in Holistic Health, Metaphysics, Parapsychology, and Divinity.

In addition, she is trained in several Traditional and Western Reiki traditions, and holds separate certification in Hypnotherapy, Flower Essences, Massage and Bodywork practices, and is a certified Yoga instructor. She is an ordained minister, Licensed Spiritual Health Coach, and Nutritional Coach and lead service provider of The Aruna Center.

A cooking enthusiast, she enjoys discovering new gluten-free and vegan recipes. She is the author of nine cookbooks at present, with more in the works.

35622103R00101

Printed in Great Britain
by Amazon